HAEMOSTATIC FAILURE IN LIVER DISEASE

DEVELOPMENTS IN HEMATOLOGY AND IMMUNOLOGY

Other titles in this series:

Lijnen, H.R., Collen, D. and Verstraete, M., eds: Synthetic Substrates in Clinical Blood Coagulation Assays. 1980. ISBN 90-247-2409-0

Smit Sibinga, C.Th., Das, P.C. and Forfar, J.O., eds: Paediatrics and Blood Transfusion. 1982. ISBN 90-247-2619-0

Fabris, N., ed: Immunology and Ageing. 1982. ISBN 90-247-2640-9

Hornstra, G.: Dietary Fats, Prostanoids and Arterial Thrombosis. 1982. ISBN 90-247-2667-0

Smit Sibinga, C.Th., Das, P.C. and Loghem, van J.J., eds: Blood Transfusion and Problems of Bleeding. 1982. ISBN 90-247-3058-9

Dormandy, J., ed: Red Cell Deformability and Filterability. 1983. ISBN 0-89838-578-4

Smit Sibinga, C.Th., Das, P.C. and Taswell, H.F., eds: Quality Assurance in Blood Banking and Its Clinical Impact. 1984. ISBN 0-89838-618-7

Besselaar, A.M.H.P. van den, Gralnick, H.R. and Lewis, S.M., eds: Thromboplastin Calibration and Oral Anticoagulant Control. 1984. ISBN 0-89838-637-3

Haemostatic Failure in Liver Disease

edited by

P. FONDU, MD

Department of Haematology, Hôpital Saint Pierre, Université Libre de Bruxelles, Brussels, Belgium

O. THIJS, MD

Department of Gastroenterology, Hôpital Saint Pierre, Université Libre de Bruxelles, Brussels, Belgium

1984 **MARTINUS NIJHOFF PUBLISHERS**
a member of the KLUWER ACADEMIC PUBLISHERS GROUP
BOSTON / THE HAGUE / DORDRECHT / LANCASTER

Distributors

for the United States and Canada: Kluwer Boston, Inc., 190 Old Derby Street, Hingham, MA 02043, USA
for all other countries: Kluwer Academic Publishers Group, Distribution Center, P.O.Box 322, 3300 AH Dordrecht, The Netherlands

Library of Congress Cataloging in Publication Data

Main entry under title:

Haemostatic failure in liver disease.

(Developments in hematology and immunology)
Includes index.
1. Blood--Coagulation, Disorders of--Congresses.
2. Liver--Diseases--Complications and sequelae--
Congresses. I. Fondu, P. II. Thijs, O. III. Series.
RC647.C55H35 1984 616.1'57 84-1685
ISBN 0-89838-640-3

ISBN 0-89838-640-3 (this volume)
ISBN 90-247-2432-5 (series)

Copyright

PRINTED IN THE NETHERLANDS

CONTENTS

Discussion from the symposium Hemostatic Failure in Liver Disease, Brussels, Belgium, 12 March 1983 has been added after each relevant chapter.

LIST OF CONTRIBUTORS

Adjizian, J.C., Central Laboratory of Haematology, CHU de Reims, Hôpital Robert Debré, Rue Alexis Carrel, 52090 Reims Cedex, France

Boer, de - van den Berg, M.A.G.,Rijksuniversiteit Limburg, Faculty of Medicine Biochemistry, P.O. Box 616, 6200 MD MAASTRICHT, The Netherlands

Büller, H.R., Department of Haematology, Division of Haemostasis, University Hospital "Wilhelmina Gasthuis", 2e Helmerstraat 106, 1054 CN AMSTERDAM, The Netherlands

Capel, P., Department of Haematology, Hôpital Universitaire St. Pierre (ULB) Rue Haute 322, B-1000 Bruxelles, Belgium

Cate, ten, J.W., Department of Haematology, Division of Haemostasis, University Hospital "Wilhelmina Gasthuis", 2e Helmerstraat 106, 1054 CN AMSTERDAM, The Netherlands

Collen, D., Department of Medical Research, KUL, Campus Gasthuisberg, Herestraat 49, B-3000 Leuven, Belgium

Crossley, I.R., King's College Hospital Medical School, University of London, Denmark Hill, London SE5 8RX, United Kingdom

Decorps Declere, A., Hôpital Paul Brousse, Unité de Chirurgie Hépato-Biliaire et Groupe de Recherche de Chirurgie Hépatique, (INSERM-U17), 94804 Villejuif Cedex, France

Drouble, C., Central Laboratory of Haematology, CHU de Reims, Hôpital Robert Debré, Rue Alexis Carrel, 51090 Reims Cedex, France

Etienne, J.C., Central Laboratory of Haematology, CHU de Reims, Hôpital Robert Debré, Rue Alexis Carrel, 51090 Reims Cedex, France

Fondu, P., Department of Haematology, Hôpital Universitaire St. Pierre (ULB), Rue Haute 322, B-1000 Bruxelles, Belgique

Franco, D., Hôpital Paul Brousse, Unité de Chirurgie Hépato-Biliaire et Groupe de Recherche de Chirurgie Hépatique, (INSERM-U17), 94804 Villejuif Cedex, France

Giddings, J.C., Department of Haematology, University Hospital of Wales, Heath Park, Cardiff CF4 4XN, United Kingdom

Gips, C.H., University of Groningen, Haematology Department, Internal Medicine, Oostersingel 59, 9713 EZ GRONINGEN, The Netherlands

Groote, de, J., Department of Medical Research, KUL, Campus Gasthuisberg, Herestraat 49, B-3000 Leuven, Belgium

Haagsma, E., University of Groningen, Haematology Department, Internal Medicine, Oostersingel 59, 9713 EZ GRONINGEN, The Netherlands

Imhoff, van, G.W., University of Groningen, Haematology Department, Internal Medicin
Oostersingel 59, 9713 EZ GRONINGEN, The Netherlands

Krom, R.A.F., University of Groningen, Haematology Department, Internal Medicine, Oostersingel 59, 9713 EZ GRONINGEN, The Netherlands

Lehn, E., Central Laboratory of Haematology, CHU de Reims, Hôpital Robert Debré, Rue Alexis Carrel, 51090 Reims Cedex, France

Lirzon, P., Central Laboratory of Haematology, CHU de Reims, Hôpital Robert Debré, Rue Alexis Carrel, 51090 Reims Cedex, France

Mannucci, P.M., Hemophilia and Thrombosis Centre, A. Bianchi Bonomi, Via Pace 15, I-20122 Milano, Italy

Masure, R., Unité d'Hémostase, Université Catholique de Louvain, Cliniques Universitaires St. Luc, 10, Avenue Hippocrate, B-1200 Bruxelles, Belgique

Pignon, B., Central Laboratory of Haematology, CHU de Reims, Hôpital Robert Debré, Rue Alexis Carrel, F-51090 Reims Cedex, France

Potron, G., Central Laboratory of Haematology, CHU de Reims, Hôpital Robert Debré, Rue Alexis Carrel, F-51090 Reims Cedex, France

Poynard, A., Central Laboratory of Haematology, CHU de Reims, Hôpital Robert Debré, Rue Alexis Carrel, F-51090 Reims Cedex, France

Reding, P., Clinic of Gastroenterology, Hôpital Universitaire St. Pierre (ULB), Rue Haute 322, B-1000 Brussels, Belgium

Roncaglioni, M.C., Instituto di Ricerche, Farmacologiche 'Mario Negri', Via Eritrea I-20157 Milan, Italy

Samama, M., Central Laboratory of Haematology, Hôtel Dieu, 1, Place du Parvis Notre Dame, F-75181 Paris Cedex 4, France

Schipper, H.G., Department of Haematology, Division of Haemostasis, University Hospital "Wilhelmina Gasthuis", 2e Helmerstraat 106, 1054 CN AMSTERDAM, The Netherlands

Smadja, C., Hôpital Paul Brousse, Unité de Chirurgie Hépato-Biliaire et Groupe de Recherche de Chirurgie Hépatique, (INSERM-U17), F-94804 Villejuif Cedex, France

Smit Sibinga, C.Th., University of Groningen, Haematology Department, Internal Medicine, Oostersingel 59, 9713 EZ GRONINGEN, The Netherlands

Soria, C., Laboratory Ste Marie, Hôtel Dieu, 1, Place du Parvis Notre Dame, F-75181 Paris Cedex 04, France

Soria, J., Laboratory Ste Marie, Hôtel Dieu, 1 Place du Parvis Notre Dame, F-75181 Paris Cedex 04, France

Soute, B.A.M., Rijksuniversiteit Limburg, Faculty of Medicine, Biochemistry, P.O. Box 616, 6200 MD MAASTRICHT, The Netherlands

Thijs, O., Clinic of Gastroenterology, Hôpital Universitaire St. Pierre (ULB), Rue Haute 322, B-1000 Brussels, Belgium

Vermeer, C., Rijksuniversiteit Limburg, Faculty of Medicine, Biochemistry, P.O. Box 6 6200 MD MAASTRICHT, The Netherlands

Wesenhagen, H., University of Groningen, Haematology Department, Internal Medicine,
Oostersingel 59, 9713 EZ GRONINGEN, The Netherlands
Williams, R., King's College Hospital Medical School, University of London,
Denmark Hill, London SE5 8RX, United Kingdom

INTRODUCTION

J. DE GROOTE

One of the most ominous and troublesome complications of the liver disease is the appearance of hemorrhagic phenomena. Many careful clinical observations about the relationship of liver function and of biliary tree pathology have been published. A vast amount of research work has been devoted to the subject. The severity of the hemorrhagic disorder is usually in relation to the liver disease. In mild chronic hepatitis or short lasting obstruction slight subcutaneous or mucosal bleeding may draw the attention of the patient and the doctor, but they are as such far from dangerous. However in acute hepatic insufficiency, in biliary cirrhosis the bleeding tendency is to be considered as a life threatening complication in about half of the cases. Moreover coagulation disturbances aggravate bleeding not only from ruptured oesophageal or gastric varices but also from gastritis or peptic ulcer. Menometrorrhagia, epistaxis and gingival bleeding may be very troublesome in these conditions. The use of diagnostic procedures such as liver puncture biopsy and peritoneoscopy are often impossible when platelets and prothrombine time are too low. In order to overcome this difficulty a procedure has been worked out taking a biopsy through a transjugular catheter placed in the hepatic vein. If a bleeding from the liver occurs it will be in the circulatory system and not cause any trouble. The operator should well be aware not to perforate the liver capsule with the needle because in that event the bleeding risk becomes again external.

Not only diagnosis, but also surgical interventions may become dangerous when hemostasis is endeavered. In some cases when either diagnostic or surgical intervention are imperative the bleeding tendency may be decreased by the administration of thrombocytes and clotting factors: 1000 ml of fresh frozen plasma may provide an adequate amount.Unfortunately they disappear rather rapidly from circulation so that about 200 ml have to be administered every 4 h in order to maintain a sufficient level. Platelets may be restored with thrombocytes enriched plasma. An infusion of an adequate amount (e.g. thrombocytes from 1000 ml of blood) should be given during the intervention and repeated as long as necessary every 24 h.

The relationship between liver and hemostasis is a vital one since the hepatocytes have to synthetise most, if not all, of the proteins which play an important role in the blood clotting process. Fortunately the liver has an overcapacity as to its synthetic function in contrast to its secretory function. Long before hemostatic failure jaundice will appear as a dominant symptom.

In many cases low levels of serum proteins especially albumin and clotting factors have been ascribed to anabolic disturbances. In a number of cases this defect was not due to a metabolic dysfunction but to a grossly deficient uptake of amino acids. The origin of this trouble appeared to be, practically always, from nutritional origin which was the consequence as well of bad feeding habits and chronic alcoholism as produced by dietary restrictions imposed by the physician. The latter, especially the family doctor, has to be fully aware of all the consequences of his advice a.o. price, social acceptability and palatability.

The level of vitamin K and the pathway dependent on it, may become insufficient in liver diseases and cause a hemostatic deficiency. The absorption of this liposoluble vitamin is partly regulated by bile excretion: its defect in longer lasting chronic obstruction is well known. In human plasma 4 clotting factors depend on the integrety of this system: factor VII, Stuart and Christmas factor and prothrombin. Their synthesis isdeficient either when the vitamin K is lacking or the synthetic pathways are blocked. In liver diseases the synthesis of precursor polypeptides seems to be impaired. In contrast polypeptide chains that lack clotting properties can be detected immunologically in vitamin K deficiency which prevents only the formation of functionally active substances. In the last circumstances the administration of vitamin K will be of clinical help. When a patient does

not readily respond to vitamin K, its administration should not be prolonged because it may be toxic when used in large amounts.
The proaccelerin or factor V deficiency is the next most common coagulation disorder in liver diseases. This factor is synthetised mostly if not exclusively in the hepatocytes. This defect only occurs in the late stages of acute and chronic pathology. It is an ominous event and the decrease of this factor may be accelerated by excessive plasma proteolytic activity and/or intravascular coagulation. A long one-stage prothrombin time reflects the low circulation level of the proaccelerin. This deficiency is difficult to correct because the factor disappears rather quickly as well from cold stored blood as from circulation.
Fibrinogen deficiency may result from impaired synthesis or from excessive utilisation. As for other proteins a decrease of fibrinogen synthesis is often due to an insufficient uptake of amino acids. An intrinsic hepatocytic deficiency is mostly the result of a severe acute hepatitis with wide spread multilobular necrosis. Intravascular coagulation is the most common cause of hypofibrinogenemia. The pathogenesis of this complication is rather obscure. Several types of activation of the clotting process have been proposed and probably all of them may contribute to it. The treatment of ascites with reinfusion of the ascitic fluid induces almost always a transient alteration of the coagulation state resembling intravascular coagulation. It results, however, rarely in a more profound fibrinolysis. The presence of thromboplastin in the ascites may be at the origin of these changes. Nevertheless dangerous hemorrhagic symptoms may sometimes occur and such procedures should be carefully monitored. In transient transfusion of the ascitic fluid this complication is never of major significance. The use of a permanent peritoneo-jugular shunt gives rise to many more such complications. The treatment of this complication is also very difficult. The infusion of fibrinogen does not seem to be effective. The use of low doses of heparin has been proposed. Fibrinogen titers do increase with this treatment which should only be used outside a major bleeding.
The hemorrhagic tendency in cirrhotic patients is often demonstrated by thrombocytopenia which could be due to the presence of portal hypertension and/or an increased utilisation in dissiminated intravascular

coagulation. In some cases the alcoholism itself causing the cirrhosis may also decrease the platelet production. The relation portal hypertension and thrombocytopenia is not fully understood. The classical hypothesis is an excessive removal or sequestration by the spleen. The fact that thrombocytopenia often occurs after splenectomy adds weight to this hypothesis. It should never be forgotten that thrombocytopenia may be strongly aggravated by the transfusion of platelet poor stored blood. As described above platelet enriched plasma may be infused in all circumstances when bleeding seems to occur in connection with a level below 100.000/mm^3 of platelets.

This book will certainly clarify many new aspects of the hemostatic phenomena in liver diseases.It will stimulate further research and discussion about the subject.

COAGULATION FACTORS SYNTHESIS BY THE LIVER, WITH SPECIAL REFERENCE TO FACTOR VIII AND FACTOR V.

J.C. GIDDINGS

The title of this current symposium emphasises the fact that we recognise the primary role of the liver in the synthesis of a wide range of plasma proteins, including coagulation factors. Many studies, utilising a variety of techniques, some of which are listed briefly in Table 1, have provided fundamental information for the diagnosis and treatment of hepatic disease.

Hepatic Synthesis of Coagulation Factors

METHOD		SELECTED REFERENCES
Fluorescence immunohistology		Barnhart (1960) Anderson and Barnhart (1964) Giddings et al (1975)
Tissue explant culture		Pool and Robinson (1959) Prydz (1964, 1965) Merskey and Wohl (1965)
Isolated liver perfusion		Mattii et al (1964) Olsen et al (1966) Shaw et al (1979) Owen and Bowie (1981)
Clinical observations	see:	Stormorken (1972)

There are, however, some aspects of coagulation factor synthesis which remain unclear and recent findings suggest that complex haemostatic mechanisms may be influenced by liver proteins in ways not fully evaluated at present. In this context the role of carboxylation of vitamin K dependent proteins and the nature of protein C are discussed in detail by other colleagues. Modern concepts regarding the production of non-vitamin K dependent coagulation factors, especially factor VIII and factor V are illustrated in the present paper.

The nature of factor VIII and of factor V is not fully understood at present and detailed discussion of their biochemistry is outside the scope of this presentation. Comphrehensive reviews have been published, for example by Hoyer (12) and Nesheim et al (13). Nevertheless, it is pertinent to consider some relevant features of these proteins. In particular, it is important to establish definitions for the various terms applied to components of the factor VIII molecule which may have given some confusion in recent years. Deficiencies of factor VIII occur in three well described hereditary haemorrhagic conditions. These are classical haemophilia A, von Willebrand's disease and the rare but well documented hereditary combined deficiency of factor V and factor VIII. The genetics of these disorders in which haemophilia A is X-linked whilst the others are autosomal, together with other simple laboratory features, illustrates the complex nature of the factor VIII molecule (table 11).

Factor VIII Deficiency - Clinical Syndromes

Simple laboratory features.

	Bleeding Time	Coagulant VIII VIIIC	Immuno precip. VIII VIIIR:Ag
Haemophilia	N	↓	N or ↑
von Willebrand's	↑	↓	↓ or A
Combined V/VIII	N or ↑	↓	N

For example, coagulant factor VIII, that is its activity measured in 'in vitro' clotting tests, is reduced in all three disorders but immuno-precipitable factor VIII is reduced or abnormal in von Willebrand's disease but normal or raised in the other conditions. In addition the presence or absence of an abnormal bleeding time in patients suggests that factor VIII or a component of factor VIII plays an important role in primary haemostasis. These findings are well known and have been extensively discussed in the context of the molecular structure of factor VIII. However, it remains uncertain whether the entities responsible for the defects are present on one molecule, on two separate molecules or on a non-covalent complex of the two although available evidence tends to favour the latter hypothesis. The complex nature of the factor VIII molecule has resulted in a varied nomenclature for the different components and it is important to understand the major terms used to describe each of the entities. As has already been noted, VIIIC is the term used to define procoagulant activity; VIIICAg or VIII clotting antigen is used to denote the antigenic determinants of VIIIC measured usually with homologous antisera in antibody neutralisation tests or immunoradiometric assays (IRMA). VIIIRAg or VIII related antigen is used to define the material detected with heterologous antibodies usually in electrophoresis tests or IRMA; and Ristocetin cofactor, RiCoF or von Willebrand factor, vWF, is used for the entity measured in platelet aggregation assays using Ristocetin. It is thought to represent the biological function of VIIIRAg.

Factor VIII terminology

VIIIC	-	procoagulant activity
VIIIC:Ag	-	antigenic determinants measured mainly with homologous antibodies - antibody neutralisation - immunoradiometric assay (IRMA)
VIIR:Ag	-	antigenic determinants measured mainly with heterologous antibodies - electrophoresis - IRMA
RiCoF (vWF)	-	biological function of VIIIR:Ag measured in Ristocetin assay.

Factor V does not appear to have as complex a structure as factor VIII but there are features which suggest considerable similarity between V and VIIIC. For example, their molecular weights in non-reduced form may be similar although in each case the precise molecular weight is disputed. The effects of thrombin, activated protein C and various inorganic adsorbants on the two proteins are the same and both appear to interact with phospholipid and co-operate as co-enzymes in blood coagulation mechanisms. Studies in patients with combined factor V and factor VIII deficiency support the possibility that these proteins have some biochemical hemology. A major site of synthesis of factor V is believed to be the hepatocyte but the cellular site of synthesis of VIIIC is uncertain. The main purpose of the present paper is to discuss the possible role of the liver in the synthesis of VIIIC and to present data comparing hepatic synthesis of VIIIC and VIIIRAg with that of factor V.

Comparison of Factors V and VIIIC

	V	VIIIC
mol wt :	350,000	? 85-300,000
effect of thrombin :	activated and then inactivated	activated and then inactivated
effect of activated Protein C :	inactivated	inactivated
activity in serum :	absent	absent
inorganic adsorbants :	not adsorbed	not adsorbed
interaction with phospholipid :	interacts	interacts
presence in platelets :	++	not proven
role in coagulation :	co-enzyme in activation of factor II	co-enzyme in activation of factor X
site of synthesis :	hepatocytes	uncertain
genetics :	combined deficiency of factors V and VIIIC	

Our preliminary approach to this study was to identify and localise the coagulation factor-antigens using specific antisera and conventional indirect immunofluorescence techniques. These methods confirmed the presence of factor V antigen in hepatic parenchymal cells particularly in sections of neonatal liver, although it is noteworthy that factor V was not as evident in sections of adult liver.

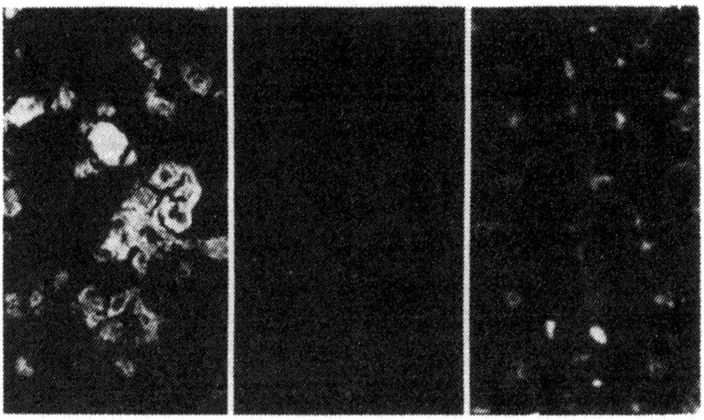

Figure 1
Immunofluorescence staining of human liver sections.
Left: neonatal liver; factor V. Centre: adult liver; factor V
Right: adult liver; factor VIIIRAg.

In contrast, similar sections treated with heterologous antifactor VIII serum, and thus detecting primarily VIIIRAg, identified positive fluorescence associated probably with cells of the hepatic sinusoids.
The results were compatible with those showing the widespread presence of VIIIRAg on the vascular endothelium, for example on the intimal surface of the hepatic artery. Subsequent studies have shown the presence of VIIIRAg on the endothelium of all human blood vessels and have demonstrated synthesis of VIIIRAg by endothelial cells in culture. (Figure 2).

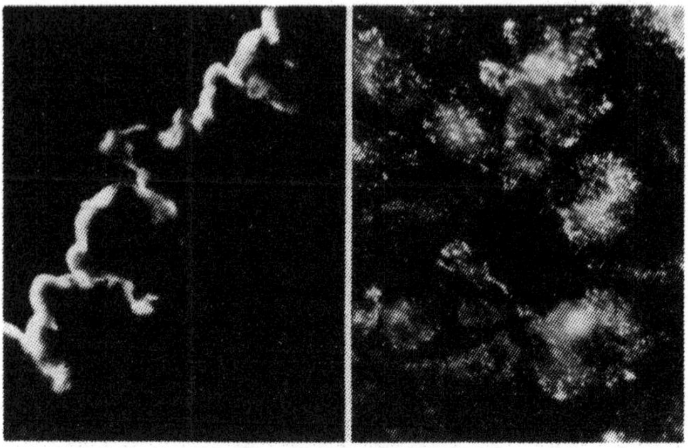

Figure 2
Immunofluorescence staining for factor VIII related antigen. Left:- adult human hepatic artery. Right:- human umbilical vein cells in culture.

Incidently, factor V antigen was observed on the intimal surface of some blood vessels (figure 3) but this was removed by washing or perfusion and was not present in cultured endothelial cells.

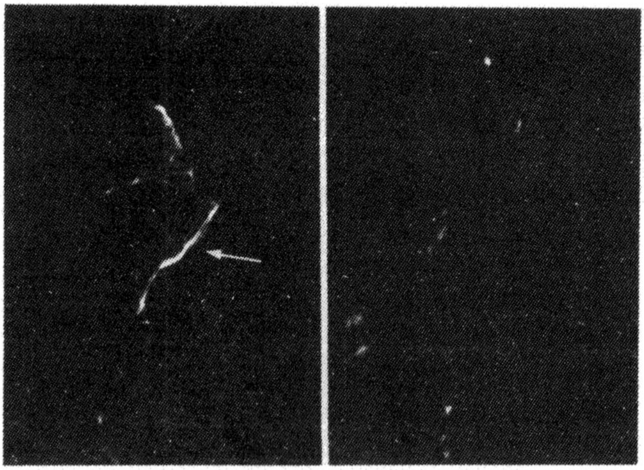

Figure 3
Immunofluorescence staining for factor V. Left: human coronary artery. Right: same artery perfused with buffer containing EDTA.

Unfortunately, it was not possible to identify VIIIC with certainty using this technique. Homologous antisera, which are believed to be specific for VIIIC gave negative or non-specific reactions with all tissues examined.

We have investigated, therefore, the hepatic synthesis of VIIIC, using an isolated organ perfusion system. Figure 4 shows a photograph of the perfusion apparatus and illustrates diagramatically the fluid circuit. In outline, perfusion fluid, of defined composition, was stirred in a central reservoir and was pumped through a heat exchange unit at 37°C into a secondary reservoir. This smaller chamber allowed removal of air bubbles from the circuit and acted to control flow to the liver by gravity pressure. At this point the fluid that was not perfused through the liver was directed through a glass, thin film oxygenator and then back to the central reservoir. Oxygenation with humidified 95% oxygen, 5% carbon dioxide was performed at several points in the circuit.

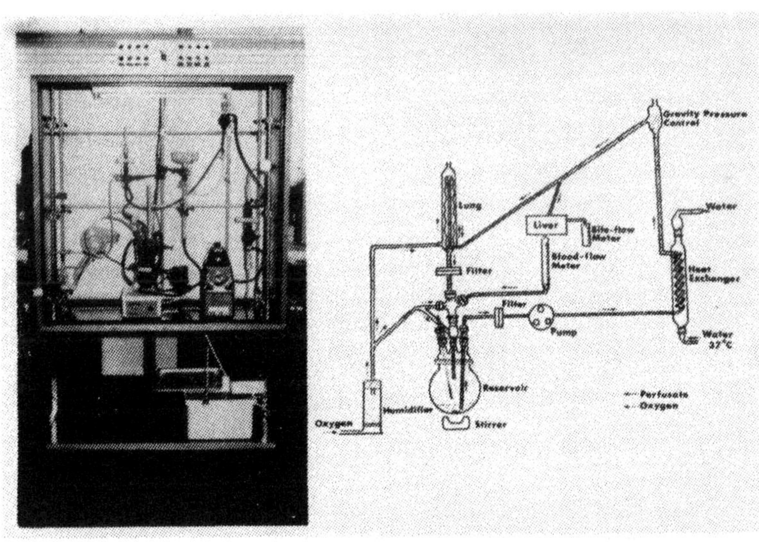

Figure 4
Photograph (left) and diagrammatic illustration (right) of isolated organ perfusion apparatus.

Livers were isolated and removed surgically from albino male Wistar rats in a rapid operative procedure designed to minimise the period of hepatic anoxia. The liver was without blood or perfusate flow for a maximum of three minutes. After removal from the animal the liver was perfused initially with recirculating fluid for 60 minutes to reduce the effect on subsequent assays of stored coagulation factors. This first fluid, termed the 'flush', was then replaced with fresh perfusion fluid and circulated for a further 180 minutes. During this time samples were removed from the main reservoir at selected intervals and replaced with an equivalent volume of fresh medium.

The basal perfusion medium consisted of carefully washed rat erythrocytes suspended in Tyrodes solution containing 0.01M sodium citrate and 3.5% bovine serum albumin. Previous experiments had determined that the presence of rat platelets and leukocytes resulted in high levels of factor V in the perfusion fluid and prevented evaluation of subsequent factor V-synthesis. Using carefully prepared erythrocyte suspensions no coagulation activity could be determined in the basal medium.

Various supplements were added to the medium to determine their effect on protein synthesis. These are given in Table V.

Additives to Basal Perfusion Medium

Protein synthesis inhibitors:			
	Actinomycin D	-	1mg per litre
	Cycloheximide	-	50mg per litre
Vitamin K antagonist:			
	Warfarin	-	12.5mg per litre
Reticulo-endotheilial blockade:			
	Amorphous carbon (Indian ink)		0.6ml i.v.
	Ethionine	-	0.001M
Radiolabelled amino acid:			
	^{35}S L- Methionine		300 µCi.

Actinomycin D, 1mg per litre and cycloheximide, 50mg per litre were added as established protein synthesis inhibitors. Warfarin, 12.5mg per litre was added as a vitamin K antagonist. In each case the additive was included in the initial flush and in the final perfusion fluid. In some experiments 0.001M DL-ethionine was added to the flush perfusate or indian ink was administered intravenously to the animal 15 minutes before sugical removal of the liver in order to block reticulo-endothelial cell function.

Some experiments were undertaken with the addition of radiolabelled methionine to the perfusate. These were performed to investigate de novo protein synthesis by assessing the inccrporation of labelled amimo acid into the perfusion product as will be described later.

Criteria for the maintenance of adequate perfusion were established to permit valid analysis of subsequent fractions. Macroscopically the liver maintained a normal appearance throughout the experiment and flow rates through the organ of greater than 10ml per minute were constant. Continuous production of bile, consumption of oxygen and maintenance of a physiological pH were also essential requisites.

Preliminary experiments were carried out to ensure that the perfusion model did indeed synthesise protein. Samples taken from perfusions in the presence of radiolabelled methionine were analysed by two dimensional crossed immunoelectrophoresis against anti rat serum followed by autoradiography. Figure 5 illustrates that both the number of precipitin lines and the strength of reaction observed on autoradiography increased with time of perfusion. Conversely, no such development occurred if the perfusion fluid contained also cycloheximide.

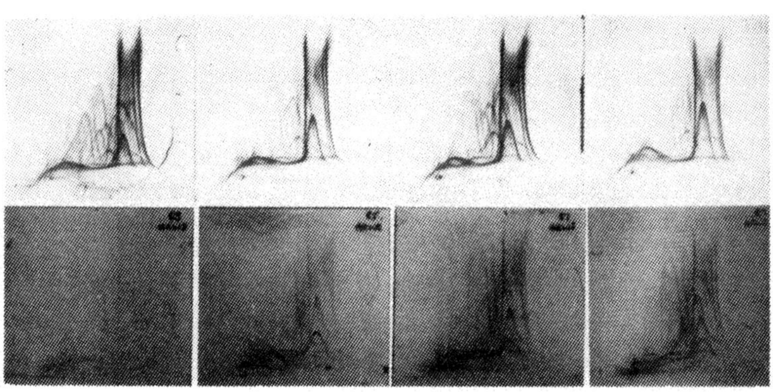

Figure 5
Two dimensional crossed immunoelectrophoresis (top sections) and corresponding autoradiographs (bottom sections) of perfusion samples taken at intervals during the final perfusion period using basal medium containing radiolabelled methionine. Perfusion time increases from left to right. 15 minutes, 60 minutes, 120 minutes, 180 minutes respectively.
Normal rat serum added to the test sample immediately before electrophoresis.

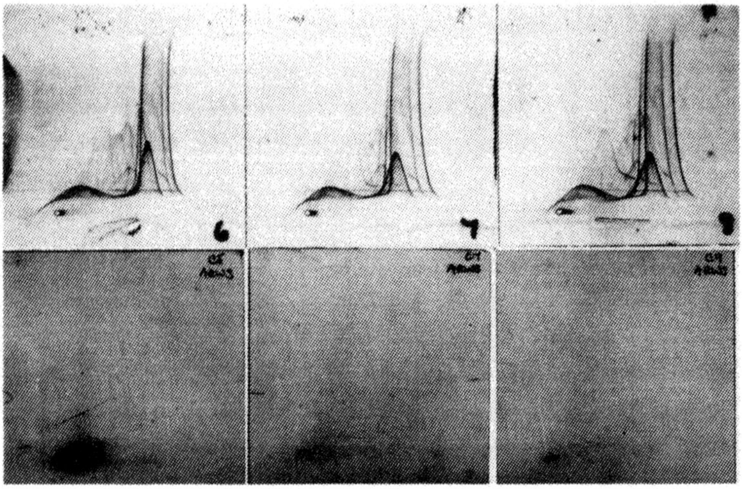

Figure 6
Two dimensional crossed immunoelectrophoresis (top) and autoradiographs (bottom) of perfusion samples taken during perfusion with medium containing radiolabelled methionine and cycloheximide. Perfusion time from left to right, 120 minutes, 180 minutes.

The precipitin lines noted on the stained immunoelectrophoresis plate are due to the addition of carrier, normal rat serum to the samples immediately before electrophoresis.

These samples and others from perfusions without radiolabelled aminacid were assayed for coagulation factor activity using conventional clotting techniques and for VIIIRAg using an IRMA for human VIIIRAg that cross-reacted with the rat protein. A reference standard for the rat coagulation factors was unavailable and the results of the clotting assays are expressed as shortening of the clotting time in seconds in the respective functional method.

Figure 7 illustrates the results of factor X assays on the various perfusion samples.

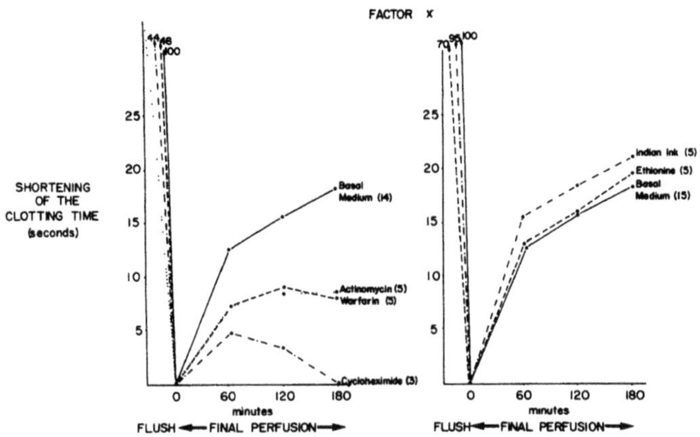

<u>Figure 7</u>
The synthesis of factor X during perfusion. The results are expressed as mean shortening of the assay clotting times (see text) The figures in parenthesis indicate the number of perfusions performed with the respective perfusion medium.

Similar results were obtained also for factor II and factor IX. The assay clotting times progressively shortened in perfusions with basal medium indicating increasing levels of coagulation factor activity. In the presence of actinomycin, cycloheximide and Warfarin the coagulation factor activity was markedly reduced. Cycloheximide had the most pronounced effect and the results are compatible with the known action of these protein synthesis inhibitors. Conversely the administration of indian ink or ethionine did not effect synthesis of factor II, IX or X.

The results of factor V assays are shown in Figure 8.

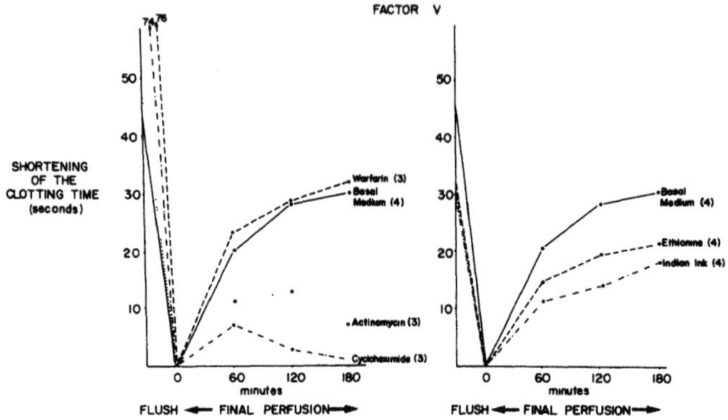

Figure 8
The synthesis of factor V during perfusion.
Actinomycin and cycloheximide had the same effect as that noted previously but Warfarin was not inhibitory. In addition, and in contrast to the results observed earlier, the injection of indian ink or inclusion of ethionine in the perfusion medium reduced the synthesis of factor V suggesting that reticulo-endothelial blockade modified the production of this protein. These results tend to contrast with the earlier immunofluorescence findings and those of other workers which suggested that factor V was synthesised by hepatic parenchymal cells. The reasons for this are not clear at present and are being investigated further. Significantly, very similar results were obtained with assays of VIIIC (Figure 9) tending to emphasise similarity between these two clotting factors.

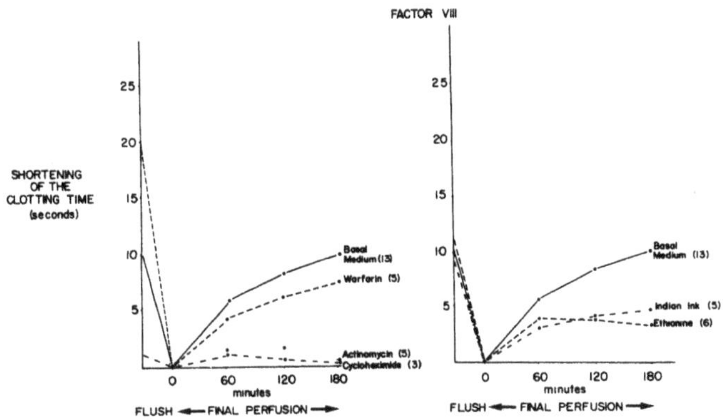

<u>Figure 9</u>
The synthesis of factor VIIIC during perfusion.

In order to confirm the site of damage caused by indian ink sections of liver were examined histologically after perfusion (Figure 10)

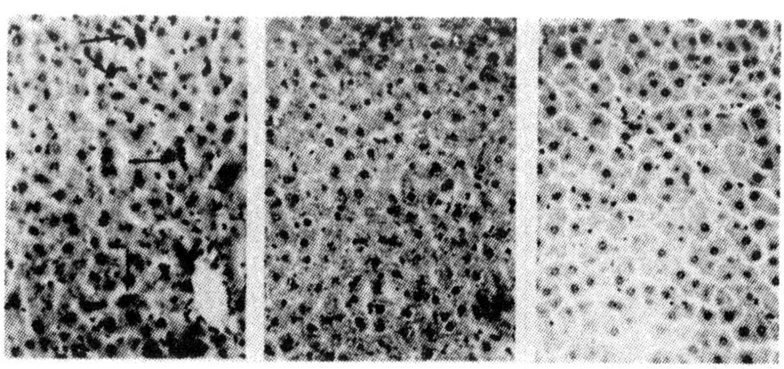

<u>Figure 10</u>
Histological appearances of rat liver after perfusion. (Haematoxylin and eosin stained sections) Left: perfusion after injection of indian ink. note the carbon particles arrowed. Centre: perfusion with basal medium. Right: perfusion with medium containing cycloheximide.

Carbon particles were confined to cells of the hepatic sinusoids presumably phagocytic reticulo-endothelial cells and the remaining cellular architecture retained a normal appearance. For comparison Figure 10 also shows the effect on liver microstructure after perfusion with basal medium and fluid containing cycloheximide. In the absence of additive there was dilatation of the liver sinusoids but little cell damage and minimal interstitial haemorrhage. In the presence of cycloheximide, pyknotic nuclei and necrotic cells were evident and there were large areas of interstitial haemorrhage. These results identified the different sites of action of the substances added to the basal perfusion medium.

To investigate further the hepatic synthesis of factor VIII, VIIICAg assays were attempted using a human inhibitor in an IRMA. Regrettably the inhibitor did not appear to cross react well with rat factor VIII in this assay system and the results were equivocal. Nevertheless, clotting times in conventional coagulation assays on perfusion samples incubated with the human inhibitor were markedly longer than those performed in the absence of inhibitor (Table V1) confirming specifically the synthesis of VIIIC.

Inhibition of Synthesised VIIIC by Human Inhibitor

	Clotting time (s) in VIIIC assay (APTT method)	
Perfusion time (min)	Medium + buffer (n = 4)	Medium + human inhibitor (n = 4)
Flush	88	122
0	126	136
60	106	130
120	100	121
180	98	122

In contrast, an IRMA for VIIIRAg, using an anti human VIIIRAg serum, demonstrated adequate cross-reactivity with rat plasma and enabled sensitive quantitation of this material. Table V11 shows that VIIIRAg was released into the perfusate but there was no significant difference between the results in the presence or absence of cycloheximide. It was not possible, therefore to demonstrate de novo synthesis of VIIIRAg in this system.

Immunoradiometric assay of VIII RAg

Perfusion time (min)	Factor VIII RAg (units/100ml; mean ± SD) Basal Medium (n = 12)	Medium + cycloheximide (n = 9)
Flush	0.87 ± 0.76	0.73 ± 0.88
0	0.01	0.02
60	0.08 ± 0.08	0.09 ± 0.07
120	0.25 ± 0.22	0.18 ± 0.15
180	0.27 ± 0.30	0.21 ± 0.15

No statistically significant difference between results of perfusion with or without cycloheximide.

From these results it appeared reasonable to suggest that the liver synthesised relatively more VIIIC than VIIIRAg. It is also possible that VIIIRAg which is synthesised and released by endothelial cells throughout the body is activated to form VIIIC or stimulates its production in the liver. To test this hypothesis Owen and his colleagues (10) perfused isolated porcine livers with blood from pigs with von Willebrand's disease and showed that VIIIC was not synthesised unless purified VIIIRAg was added. In the present study perfusions were also undertaken in the presence of exogenous VIIIRAg. Purified protein from human and rat plasma was added to the basal medium in graded concentrations and VIII related assays performed in the usual way. In all instances VIIIRAg consistently decreased in the perfusion fluid, confirming the report of Owen and his co-workers.

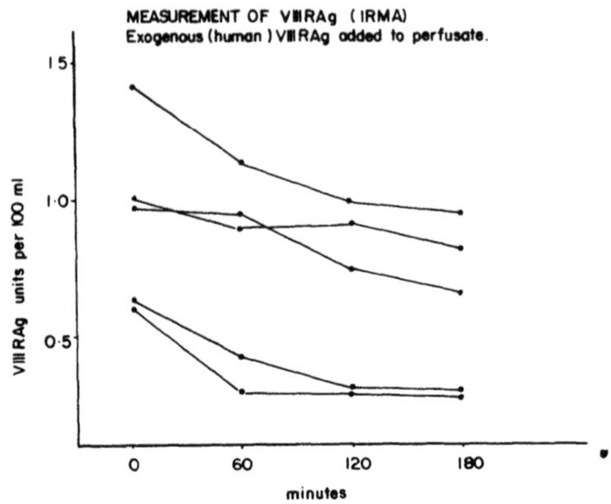

Figure 11
Decrease in VIIIRAg concentrations during perfusion.

However, the synergistic effect on VIIIC synthesis noted by Owen was not observed in our studies. On the contrary, the results tended to show inhibition of VIIIC production in the presence of exogenous VIIIRAg.

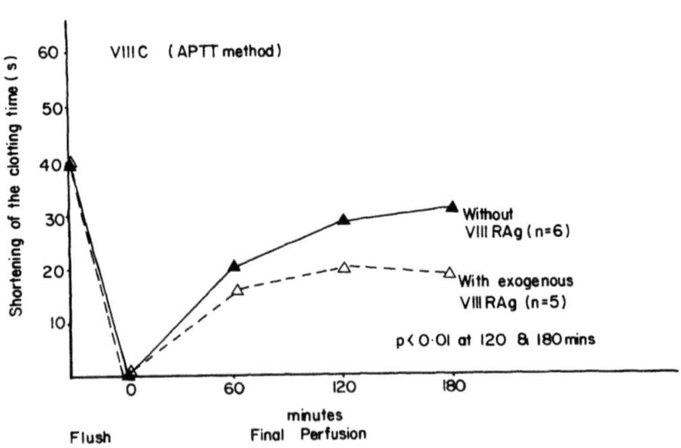

Figure 12
The effect of exogenous human VIIIRAg on the synthesis of VIIIC during perfusion.

Nevertheless, the results emphasised a significant role for the liver in the synthesis or modification of components of the factor VIII molecule and this remains to be fully evaluated.

In conclusion, therefore, immunohistological studies and isolated organ perfusion techniques have demonstrated hepatic localisation and synthesis of coagulation factors II, IX, X, V and VIIIC. Synthesis of V and VIIIC was inhibited by actinomycin and cycloheximide in a manner similar to that observed with factors II, IX and X and was not inhibited by Warfarin. The cells which synthesise V and VIIIC are susceptable to ethionine and indian ink suggesting possible reticulo-endothelial cell origins. Relatively more VIIIC than VIIIRAg was synthesised in the isolated liver perfusion system and exogenous VIIIRAg was consistently removed from the circulating perfusate. In spite of extensive efforts the precise cellular sites of synthesis of V and VIIIC remains to be established. Application of modern technology, for example using monoclonal antibodies, may help to clarify the role of the liver in the production of these clinically important plasma proteins.

ACKNOWLEDGEMENTS

A substantial part of the work described in this presentation was undertaken by Mrs. E. Shaw in collaboration with Professor. A.L. Bloom. We are grateful to the editor and publishers of The British Journal of Haematology for permission to reproduce previously published figures. The work was supported by grants from the Arthritis and Rheumatism Council and The Medical Research Council.

REFERENCES

1. Barnhart, M.I 1960 Cellular site for prothrombin synthesis. American Journal of Physiology, 199, 360
2. Anderson, G.F and Barnhart, M.I, 1966. Prothrombin synthesis in the dog. American Journal of Physiology, 206, 929.
3. Giddings, J.C., Shearn, S.A.M., Bloom, A.L., 1975 The immunological localisation of factor V in human tissue. British Journal of Haematolog 29, 57.
4. Pool, J.G., Robinson, J, 1959. In vitro synthesis of coagulation factors by rat liver slices. American Journal of Physiology, 196, 423.
5. Prydz, H. 1964. Studies on proconvertin (factor VII). Biosynthesis in suspension cultures of rat liver cells. Scandinavian Journal of Clinical and Laboratory Investigation, 16, 540.
6. Merskey, C., Wohl, H 1965. In vitro production of coagulation factors VII and X by liver slices from rats fed atherogenic diets. Proceedings of the Society for Experimental Biology and Medicine. 118, 703.
7. Mattii, R., Ambrus, J.L., Sokal, I.E., Mink, E. 1964. Production of members of the blood coagulation and fibrinolysis systems by the isolated perfused liver. Proceedings of the Society for Experimental Biology and Medicine. 116, 69.
8. Olson, J.P., Miller, L.L., Troup, S.B 1966. Synthesis of clotting factors by the isolated perfused rat liver. Journal of Clinical Investigation, 45, 690.
9. Shaw, E., Giddings, J.C., Peake, I.R., Bloom, A.L 1979. Synthesis of procoagulant factor VIII, factor VIII related antigen and other coagulation factors by the isolated perfused rat liver. British Journal of Haematology, 41, 585.
10. Owen, C.A., Bowie, E.J.W. 1981. Generation of plasmatic coagulation factors by the isolated rat liver perfused with completely synthetic blood substitute. Thrombosis Research, 22, 259.
11. Stormorken, H. 1973. Editor. Proceedings of a symposium on coagulation and liver disease. Scandinavian Journal of Gastroenterology. 8, Supplement 19.
12. Hoyer, L.W 1981. The factor VIII complex: Structure and function. Blood, 58, 1.
13. Nesheim, M.E., Katzmann, J.A., Tracy, P.B., Mann, K.G. 1981. Factor V in Methods in Enzymology. Proteolytic Enzymes. Editor L. Lorand. pp 249-274. Academic Press, New York.

DISCUSSION LECTURE GIDDINGS

Burmane Do you have an idea of the molecular weight of FVIII:c in your experiments?

Giddings No, the level is so low that it is impossible to do any chromatography or anything of that nature on the perfusion samples. As it happens, incidentally, the studies that we have done on FVIII:c molecular weight with other methods, have tended a conflict with what other people said and we are not very happy with our methodology at the moment, so we have not gone into that area yet. But the reported molecular weights varies between 25 and 300.000 for the intact molecule anyway.

Question from the audience

Giddings I do not know. I suspect that the liver is not the only site of synthesis, that's all I can say. I would be very surprised if that sort of cell specifically in the liver would produce FVIII:c. For other physiological reasons, for example the release of FVIII:c when you give DDAVP, which is so instantanious and so potent that I would be very surprised if it attacks that target side like that in the liver. But I think that remains to be seen.

Vinnazer You don't have normal levels of coagulation factors in rats so how did you make you calibration curve?

Giddings Yes, we did not have a reference material, we did not have a reference standards in rats; what we did, was to pool a lot of rat plasma and to use that to relate to humans. We were unhappy about calling it a quantitated value in the assay; simply we have just shorten the clotting time. But we were getting calibration curves with normal pooled rat plasma.

ORAL ANTICOAGULANTS: UNEXPECTED SIDE-EFFECTS OR NEW FIELDS OF APPLICATION?

MARIAN A.G. DE BOER-V.D. BERG, M. CARLA RONCAGLIONI,[+] BERRY A.M. SOUTE, MENNO DE METZ AND CEES VERMEER[*]

1. SUMMARY

Vitamin K-dependent carboxylase is found in liver and in a number of non-hepatic tissues such as: testis, lung, kidney, spleen and arterial vessel wall. It is shown, that the dosages of warfarin, required for a partial inhibition of the clotting factor synthesis also affects the non-hepatic vitamin K-dependent systems. The presence of non-hepatic vitamin K-dependent carboxylase is demonstrated in various rat and bovine tissues as well as in human placenta and it has to be expected, that also other human tissues contain this enzyme. Whether the inhibition of non-hepatic carboxylase, which occurs during oral anticoagulant therapy is harmful, neutral or beneficial for the patient can only be judged when the function of the various vitamin K-dependent proteins is known.

2. INTRODUCTION

It has been known for many years, that vitamin K is involved in the production of 4 blood clotting factors. These factors are all synthesized in the liver, and during their maturation they are carboxylated in a posttranslational process (1). The enzyme involved is designated as carboxylase and vitamin K functions as its coenzyme. The substrate for carboxylase is a number of glutamic acid (glu) residues in the N-terminal part of the clotting factor precursors, which are carboxylated into gammacarboxyglutamic acid (gla) residues (2). Before it can act as a

* to whom all correspondence should be addressed.

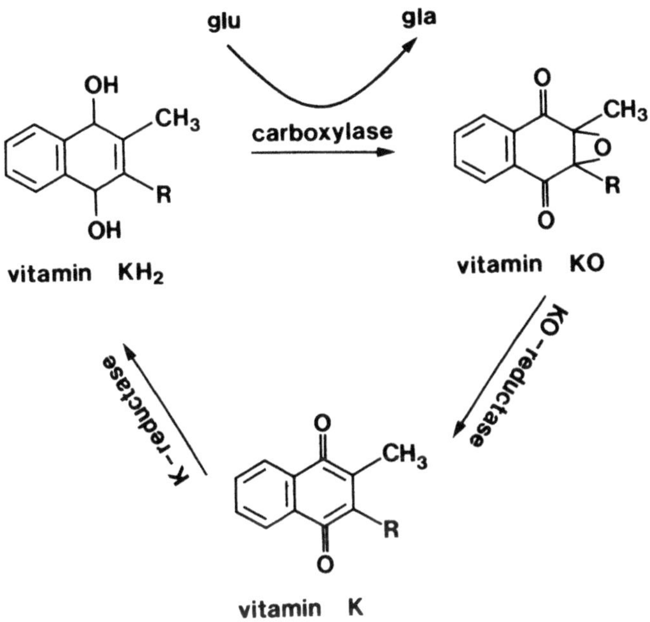

FIGURE 1. The vitamine K-cycle

coenzyme in the carboxylation reaction, vitamin K has to be transformed from the quinone form (which is the most stable form) into the more reduced hydroquinone (3). Although at this moment the evidence is not irrefutable, it is generally believed that during the carboxylation reaction vitamin K hydroquinone is oxidized and converted into vitamin K epoxide (4). The epoxide is than reduced again, either to vitamin K quinone or directly to vitamin K hydroquinone. This sequence of reactions is called the vitamin K cycle (fig.1). In this view the oxidation of vitamin K hydroquinone provides the energy for the conversion of glu into gla. Coumarin derivatives, which are frequently used as anticoagulants, inhibit the enzyme(s) involved in the reduction of vitamin K epoxide (4). During anticoagulant therapy, the epoxide therefore accumulates in the liver and the formation of normal clotting factors is reduced because the pool of vitamin K hydroquinone gets exhausted.

In this paper we give an overview of the non-hepatic tissues where vitamin K-dependent reactions take place and we try to verify whether the anticoagulant therapy affects also the non-hepatic carboxylase.

3. MATERIALS AND METHODS

Chemicals. Warfarin and dithiothreitol (DTT) were obtained from Sigma, the detergent CHAPS was from Serva and vitamin K_1 from Hoffman-La Roche. Vitamin K hydroquinone was prepared as described earlier (5). $NaH^{14}CO_3$ (40-60 Ci/mol) and Atomlight were from New England Nuclear and the synthetic substrate Phe-Leu-Glu-Glu-Leu (FLEEL) was from Vega Biochemicals. The Thrombotest reagent was purchased from Nyegaard & Co. All other chemicals were from Merck.

Methods. The rats used in some experiments were male Wistar rats of 12-15 weeks old. Warfarin (as indicated) was dissolved in 20 mM phosphate buffer, pH 9.0, which substituted for their drinking water.
Microsomes were prepared from the various rat and bovine tissues as described in (6). Carboxylase was solubilized from these preparations by adding 1.0 % CHAPS in 0.8 M NaCl. Carboxylase activity was measured by the incorporation of $^{14}CO_2$ into endogenous or exogenous substrate (FLEEL) and all results are expressed as the amount of incorporated label per mg of microsomal protein. The way in which carboxylase and the endogenous substrate are quantified is fully explained in (5).

The clotting-times of plasma were measured with the Thrombotest reagent and compared with a reference curve, which was prepared using pooled citrate plasma from 20 normal animals. The data are expressed as a percentage of the normal, e.g. 10 % means that the clotting-time of the plasma is similar to that of 10-fold diluted reference plasma.

4. RESULTS

Using the cow as an experimental model we have investigated the occurence of vitamin K-dependent carboxylase in a number of tissues. The cows were treated with warfarin (1.5 gram daily) for 6 days before they were slaughtered and the various organs were excised and used for the preparation of the microsomal fractions. The presence of carboxylase was investigated in these preparations and the results are summarized in table I. In all tissues where we were able to detect carboxylase we also observed

Table I. Relative amounts of microsomal carboxylase and endogenous substrate in various bovine tissues.

Tissue	Carboxylase	Substrate
Liver	100	100
Testis	140	90
Uterus	30	10
Kidney	70	30
Spleen	60	40
Lung	60	15
Thyroid	30	10
Pancreas	10	5
Thymus	10	5
Bone (epihysis)	25	10
Arteries	60	10
Veins	0	0
Heart muscle	0	0
Skeletal muscle	0	0
Diaphragm	0	0

The amounts of carboxylase (80 $dpm.min^{-1}.mg^{-1}$) and endogenous substrate (4000 $dpm.mg^{-1}$) in liver were arbitrarily chosen to be 100. All data are the mean values of at least 3 different animals. For further details see Materials and Methods.

that during the warfarin-treatment of the animal an endogenous substrate had accumulated in the microsomes. These endogenous substrates were not present in similar preparations from non-treated animals (data not shown). No differences between the various carboxylating systems could be found with respect to their optimal reaction conditions, the K_m of vitamin K or the warfarin concentration required for a 50% inhibition of this carboxylation reaction.

Now we knew that vitamin K-dependent carboxylase was present in many bovine tissues, the question arose, whether we could also detect this enzyme in human tissues. Since human tissues are less easily available than are tissues from animal origin, we could only test the carboxylase content of human liver and placenta. In fig. 2 the solubilized microsomes from these tissues are compared with those from bovine liver. Since the human material was from non-anticoagulated donors, it was compared with carboxylase from normal cows. The carboxylase content of placenta was about 40% of that in liver and it may be expected, also other human tissues will contain the vitamin K-dependent enzyme system. Recently, for instance, we

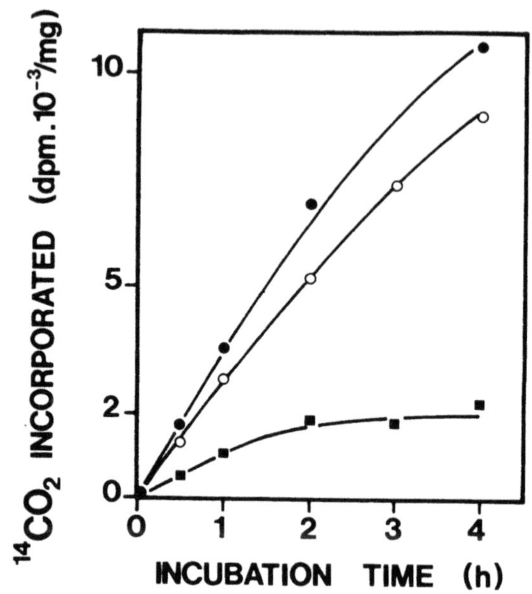

FIGURE 2. Carboxylase in human liver and placenta.
Carboxylase was measured under standard reaction conditions in the presence of 10 mM FLEEL. Carboxylase from bovine liver (●——●) is compared with that from human liver (○——○) and human placenta (■——■). Human livers were obtained from healthy donors, who died after traffic accidents and who had previously signed a donor-codicil. Carboxylase from term human placentae was prepared from the microsomal fraction of trophoblast in a similar way as was carboxylase from liver. All tissues were obtained from non-anticoagulated invididuals. Each point represents the mean value of three different donors, measured in duplicate. The carboxylation of exogenous substrate is expressed as dpm per mg of microsomal proteins.

have been able to demonstrate carboxylase in the arteries of human umbilical cord. It could be confirmed that this carboxylase was only present in the arterial vessel wall and not in that of the umbilical vein (data not shown).

In the experiments described so far we have demonstrated a) the existence of non-hepatic carboxylating enzymes and b) that these non-hepatic carboxylases are all inhibited when the experimental animals are treated with a high dose of warfarin. The warfarin is administrated in excess in order to ensure a maximal accumulation of endogenous substrates in the liver and in the other tissues. In patients, however, antivitamin K-drugs are frequently used in about 100-fold lower quantities (when expressed as mg of anticoagulant per kg body weight) and under these conditions the synthesis of the vitamin K-dependent clotting factors is only partly

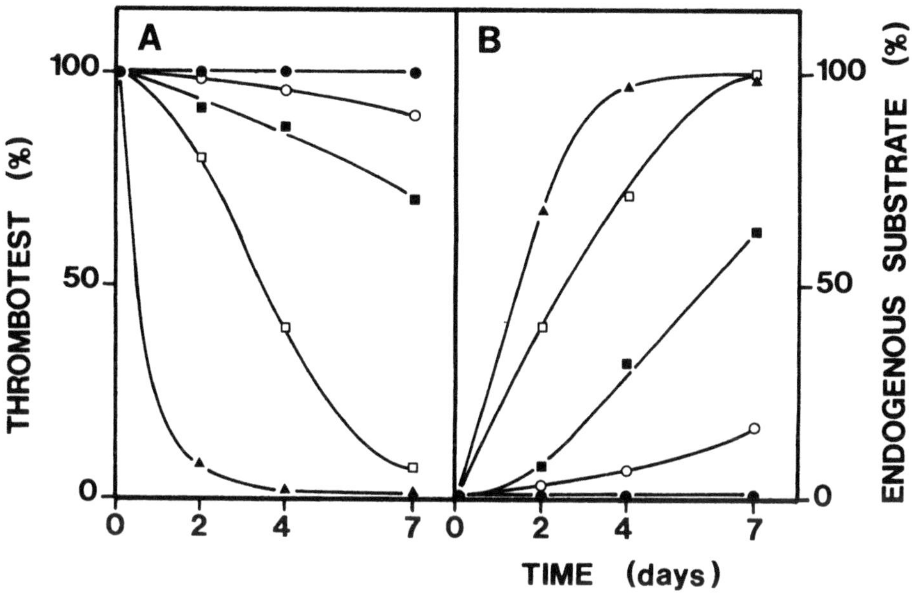

FIGURE 3. The effect of warfarin on rat liver carboxylase.
Rats were treated with warfarin, which was present in their drinking water in a concentration of: 0 mg/l (●——●), 0.5 mg/l (○——○), 1 mg/l (■——■), 2 mg/l (□——□) and 5 mg/l (▲——▲). At the indicated times three rats from each group were sacrificed and the effect of the warfarin-treatment was measured on the plasma concentration of the vitamin K-dependent clotting-factors (Thrombostest, fig 3A) and on the amount of endogenous substrate for carboxylase, present in their liver microsomes (fig 3B). The endogenous substrate is expressed as a percentage of the maximum (12,200 dpm per mg of microsomal proteins), obtained after 7 days of treatment with 2 and 5 mg/l of warfarin.

inhibited. Therefore we investigated whether these low dosages of warfarin also affect the non-hepatic carboxylases. For our experiments we needed experimental animals in larger numbers than before and therefore the rat was the animal of choice. Fourty five rats were divided into five groups of nine rats each, and warfarin was added to their drinking water in concentrations that varied from 0 in group I to 5 mg/liter in group V. The daily water intake was 20-30 ml per rat. After several intervals three rats from each group were sacrificed and the effect of the warfarin was measured in their blood plasma (fig. 3A) and in their liver (fig. 3B). Obviously the

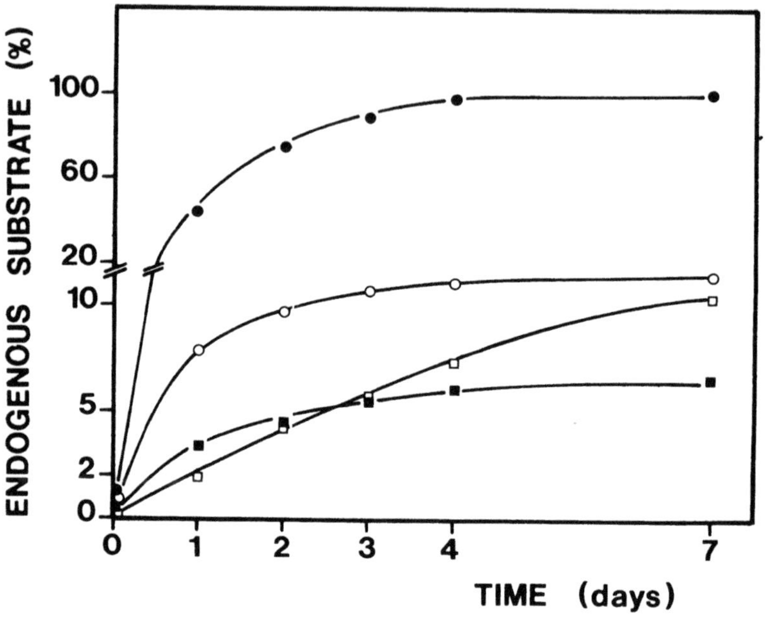

FIGURE 4. The effect of low doses of warfarin on non-hepatic tissues. The accumulation of endogenous substrates was measured under standard conditions and the results are expressed as a percentage of the amount of hepatic substrate (12,200 dpm per mg of microsomal proteins) that had accumulated after 7days of treatment with 2 mg/l of warfarin. The following tissues were examined: liver (●——●), lung (○——○), spleen (■——■), and testis (□——□).

decrease of the plasma clotting factors occurs simultaneously with the accumulation of endogenous substrate for carboxylase in the liver. At a concentration of 2 mg per liter of drinking water the warfarin only partly inhibited the hepatic carboxylase and we decided to investigate whether at that concentration also the non-hepatic carboxylases are inhibited. The warfarin was given to a group of 30 rats and after several intervals 6 rats were sacrificed and the amount of endogenous substrate was measured in the microsomal fractions of their liver, lung, spleen and testis. The results of these experiments are shown in fig. 4 and it is obvious, that also at low dosages of warfarin all non-hepatic carboxylases that were investigated were inhibited by the anticoagulant, so that endogenous substrates accumulated in the respective microsomal fractions.

5. DISCUSSION

In this paper we have demonstrated that vitamin K-dependent carboxylase is an enzyme that occurs in many different tissues. When comparing the amounts of carboxylase and endogenous substrate in these tissues, one should realize, that all data are expressed in units per mg microsomal protein. Since the total amount of microsomal proteins that can be extracted is different for each tissue, the data shown in table I are not representative for the total production of vitamin K-dependent proteins by the various organs.

It was also shown, that the non-hepatic carboxylases are inhibited under the conditions that are frequently used for the therapeutical treatment of patients (oral anticoagulant therapy). Although these results were obtained with experimental animals, there is no reason to believe that this situation is different in man. When the inhibition of the non-hepatic carboxylases is regarded as a side-effect of oral anticoagulant therapy, we have to explain why, despite of the fact that coumarin derivatives have been used on a large scale for many years, clinical symptoms of this side-effect are only hardly known. We might assume, for instance, that all vitamin K-dependent proteins are produced in great excess, so that a 90% decrease of their synthesis does not lead to clinical symptoms. On the other hand it might also be that, because we do not know the function of the non-hepatic vitamin K-dependent proteins, a number of clinical symptoms, related with the side-effects of oral anticoagulant therapy have been overlooked.

It is obvious that, before we can prove the correctness of one of these hypothesis, we will have to know the function of the non-hepatic vitamin K-dependent proteins. Unfortunately our knowledge comes to an end at this point. The proteins have been detected, some of them have even been purified and extensively characterized, but this information does not necessarily lead to the elucidation of their function. It is our opinion that for a solution of this problem a close cooperation between biochemists and clinicians is required. Because we feel that it might be helpful in diagnosing hitherto unexpected effects of coumarin derivatives on processes other than blood coagulation, we would like to discuss some of our results into more detail and to speculate about the function that some of the non-hepatic vitamin K-dependent proteins might have. Before starting these speculations, we should keep in mind that up till now the only known function of gla-residues is the strong and selective binding of Ca^{2+}. All functions described to the various gla-containing proteins should therefore be dependent of or related with the binding or the transport of Ca^{2+}.

In the first place we want to mention the striking difference between the carboxylase content of arteries and that of veins. Arterial vessel wall contains a high amount of carboxylase, whereas in veins the enzyme could not be detected. In this respect it is suggestive, that atherosclerosis occurs almost exlusively in the arteries and that a gla-containing protein (atherocalcin) has been identified in hardened atherosclerotic plaque (7). We should not exclude, therefore, the possibility that atherocalcin is involved in the calcification of the arterial vessel wall. A possible dominant role of this protein in the formation of a thrombus would be obscured by the following reasons. Patients with a high risk of thrombosis or myocardial infarction are generally kept on oral anticoagulant therapy. It has been demonstrated, that this therapy reduces the risk of reinfarction (8) and it is believed that this beneficial effect is related to the reduced plasma concentration of the vitamin K-dependent coagulation factors. Since during the anticoagulant therapy also the arterial carboxylase will be inhibited, the reduced synthesis of atherocalcin might be of greater importance than the reduced concentration of clotting factors.

A second point of interest is the high amount of carboxylase in bovine testis. We have also detected this type of carboxylase in the testis of other species and it is tempting to speculate about the function of the protein that is carboxylated by this system. Probably this protein will be a sperm protein and a logical candidate is acrosin, a trypsin-like serine protease which has many similarities with prothrombin and which is required for the penetration of the sperm chromosomes into the ovum (9). The synthesis of such a protein would be inhibited during long-term oral anticoagulant therapy, which might result in a reduced fertility of the sperm cells. Most patients, treated with vitamin K antagonists are over 50 years old and maybe this is the reason why their fertility has never been checked. At this moment we have been informed about three patients who were capable of begetting offspring after more than one year of continuous oral anticoagulant therapy. We would suggest, however, to statistically analyze the fertility of large groups of patients.

One of the best documented side-effects of coumarin derivatives is the warfarin syndrome, the abnormal bone growth in the fetus during pregnancy (10). Possibly this syndrome is due to the decreased production of osteocalcin, the gla-containing protein which is abundantly present in bone. It has been demonstrated that osteocalcin is synthesized by cultured bone cells (11), which is in agreement with the fact that we could prepare carboxylase from epiphysis. However, although the primary structure of osteocalcin has been elucidated a number of years ago, we do not know its precise function. Also no skeletal abnormalities have been reported in adults even after many years of oral anticoagulant therapy. Nevertheless it would be interesting to investigate the occurence of a number of bone-diseases under patients receiving vitamin K-antagonists. In this respect it is suggestive that in a study in 1971 of three postmenopausal patients with osteoporosis, the loss of calcium was found to be reduced 18 to 50% by daily treatment with vitamin K (12).

Finally we would like to discuss the possible function of the gla-protein produced by the kidney. Obviously the renal gla-protein may play a role in the transport and/or excretion of Ca^{2+}. Recently a gla-protein has been described that occurs in renal stones (13) and it would be interesting to know whether this protein is similar to or related with the protein, synthesized by renal carboxylase. When at some stage of the Ca^{2+} excretion a gla-protein is involved, the Ca^{2+} concentration in the kidney might increase during anticoagulant therapy, resulting in a more frequent occurrence of renal stones. On the other hand, the renal gla-proteins might also serve as nuclei for the cristallization of calcium salts. In this view the inhibition of renal carboxylase by vitamin K-antagonists would lead to a decreased production of renal gla-proteins and hence to a decreased frequency of renal stones. On beforehand neither of these two possiblities can be excluded and statistical analysis of the medical records from patients on long-term anticoagulant therapy is once more recommended.

We want to stress, that we do not expect that threatening or extremely harmful complications of the oral anticoagulant therapy will be discovered: these would have been known already for many years. However, we do hope that tendencies will be found after careful analyzis of the medical records of patients who received long-term anticoagulant therapy. The registration of these tendencies may help us in understanding the function of the non-hepatic vitamin K-dependent proteins. This knowledge might lead to a substantial extension of the processes that can be regulated by vitamin K-antagonists. The present coumarin derivatives inhibit all carboxylating systems to the same degree and it is our opinion, that new vitamin K-antagonists have to be developed, which each specifically inhibit the carboxylase present in one particular organ or tissue. This might enable us, for instance, to completely block the renal carboxylase (which may be beneficial for the patient) without simultaneously inhibiting the synthesis of clotting factors.

ACKNOWLEDGMENTS
The authors wish to thank dr. H.C. Hemker for his stimulating discussions and kindly reading this manuscript. This research was supported by grant MD 82145 from the Thrombosestichting Nederland. M.C. Roncaglioni is a recipient of the European Community Training Fellowship 1982-1983.

6. REFERENCES

1. Suttie JW, Jackson CM. 1977. Prothrombin structure, activation and biosynthesis. Phys. Rev. 57:1-70.
2. Stenflo J, Fernlund P, Egan W, Roepstorff P. 1974. Vitamin K-dependent modifications of glutamic acid residues in prothrombin. Proc. Natl. Acad. Sci. U.S.A. 71:2730-2733.
3. Olson RE, Suttie JW. 1978. Vitamin K and gamma-carboxyglutamate biosynthesis. Vitam. Horm. 35:59-108.
4. Suttie JW. 1980. Mechanism of action of vitamin K: synthesis of gammacarboxyglutamic acid. CRC Crit.Rev.Biochem. 8:191-223.
5. Vermeer C. Soute BAM, de Metz M, Hemker HC. 1982. A comparison between vitamin K-dependent carboxylase from normal and warfarin-treated cows. Biochim. Biophys. Acta 714:361-365.
6. Vermeer C, Hendrix H, Daemen M. 1982. Vitamin K-dependent carboxylases from non-hepatic tissues. FEBS Lett. 148:317-320.
7. Levy RJ, Lian JB, Gallop P. 1979. Atherocalcin, a gammacarboxyglutamic acid containing protein from atherosclerotic plaque. Biochem. Biophys. Res. Commun. 91:41-49.
8. The Sixty Plus Reinfarction Study Research Group. 1981. Lancet ii:989-994.
9. Müller-Esterl W, Fritz H. 1981 Meth. Enzymol. 80:621-632.
10. Gallop PM, Lian JB. Hauschka PV 1980. Carboxylated calcium binding proteins and vitamin K. N. Engl. J. Med. 302:1460-1466.
11. Nishimoto SK, Price PA. 1980. Secretion of the vitamin K-dependent protein of bone by rat osteosarcoma cells. J. Biol. Chem. 255:6579-6583.
12. Tomita A. 1971. Post menopausal osteoporosis ^{47}Ca study with vitamin K_2. Clin. Endocrinol. 19:731-736.

13. Lian JB, Prien EL Jr, Glimcher MJ, Gallop PM. 1977. The presence of protein-bound gamma-carboxyglutamic acid in calcium-containing renal calculi. J. Clin. Invest. 59:1151-1157.

DISCUSSION LECTURE DE BOER

Kahlé — You did not show inhibition of the carboxylation but you showed an increase in the inductionous carboxylation. Couldn't it be so that the PIVKA protein from the liver is absorbed by the other tissues and so you measure an increase in the inductionous carboxylation?

De Boer — No, in that case you find antigenicity to the clotting factors; we have looked to the nature of this substrate by immuno-specific reactions, for clotting factors, and we did not find any reaction. We don't think that that is true.

Samama — Can you evaluate easily carboxylase in man after biopsy of the liver; is it easily performed or is it difficult task? Would you suggest biopsy?

De Boer — Well, from liver it is very easy to prepare, but there is one problem: it takes a long time before we get a liver; when patient dies at least 2 hours before, we have the liver in our hands, so, in that time, maybe there can occur a lot of proteolysis and it is known that with proteolysis, also some enzymatic reactions occur.

Samama — But you cannot evaluate the activity of carboxylases on a liver biopsy?

De Boer — No, we need a large amount of liver.

Verstraete — Whether, I missed one of those, was it human or animal tissue?

De Boer — It was animal. It was from a bull calf.

Verstraete — Did you try human tissue?

De Boer — We appreciate to do that, but it is very difficult to get human tissues. If you have some for me I will be very lucky.

Samama — You said that you gave to the cow 10 mg of "Warfarin" by kg body weight, which is the dose for a human of 60 kg; it is so different.

De Boer — Well, it is a high dose, yes.

PROTEIN C, AN INHIBITOR OF BLOOD COAGULATION, IN LIVER DISEASE AND OTHER CLINICAL CONDITIONS

P.M.MANNUCCI, S.VIGANO

INTRODUCTION

In 1976 Stenflo (1) isolated from bovine plasma a new vitamin K-dependent plasma glycoprotein he called Protein C. Bovine Protein C is composed of a light chain and a heavy chain held together by disulfide bonds. The aminoterminal region of the light chain contains γ-carboxyglutamic residues, necessary for Ca^{2+} binding, as do other vitamin K-dependent coagulation proteins. In 1979 Kisiel (2) isolated and partially characterized human Protein C, with a mol. wt. of 62,000. Human and bovine Protein C appear to be remarkably similar in terms of amino acid and carbohydrate composition, with the exception of their histidine, valine and N-acetylglucosamine contents. Like other vitamin K-dependent coagulation proteins, Protein C exists in plasma in a zymogen form and is converted to a serine protease by thrombin, Russel Viper venom and trypsin. The enzyme formed, referred to as activated Protein C, has anticoagulant properties. The rate of in vitro activation of purified Protein C by thrombin is too slow to have any physiological importance. However, infusion of thrombin in dogs leads to the formation of anticoagulant activity in the circulation within 5 min after starting the infusion (3). The thrombin-catalyzed activation of Protein C is markedly accelerated in vivo by an endothelial cell surface cofactor called thrombomodulin (4,5). Recently, thrombomodulin has been purified from rabbits lungs (6). When bound to thrombomodulin, thrombin cleaves fibrinogen and factor V poorly, if at all. Therefore, the thrombin-thrombomodulin complex seems to have two distinct anticoagulant activities: it leads to direct inhibition of thrombin procoagulant activity and activates Protein C, which can then function as a circulating anticoagulant.

Mechanism of action and physiological regulation

The anticoagulant nature of activated bovine Protein C was described over 20 years ago by Seegers and his associates (7). They suggested that this potent anticoagulant activity, called autoprothrombin II-A, was derived from prothrombin that had been activated by limited thrombin proteolysis. A decade later, Marciniak (8) suggested that human autoprothrombin II-A was not derived from prothrombin but was a distinct species-specific protein. The anticoagulant activity of activated bovine Protein C was initially ascribed to a competitive inhibition of factor X_a (9, 10).

Subsequently, various investigators have shown that bovine activated protein C enzymatically inactivates bovine factors V and VIII by limited proteolysis (10, 11, 12). Marlar et al (13) have recently reported that when activated human Protein C is incubated with normal plasma phospholipid and Ca^{2+}, factor V and VIII coagulant activities are rapidly de - stroyed. Activated Protein C can inactivate activated forms of factors V and VIII more rapidly than non-activated factors. Activated Protein C has no effect on either the contact system proteins (factors XI and XII, prekallikrein and high mol.wt. kininogen) nor the vitamin K-dependent coagulation factors (prothrombin, factors VII, IX and X). No effect on fibrinogen was noted either.

In addition to its anticoagulant activity, activated Protein C has been shown (14, 15) to enhance fibrinolysis. Comp and Esmon (16) have confirmed that fibrinolytic activity can be generated both in vivo and in vitro in response to activated Protein C. The in vivo administration of small quantities of activated Protein C results in an increased rate of clot lysis. The active site of activated Protein C is necessary for the enhancement of clot lysis because neither the DFP-inhibited enzyme nor the zymogen enhance clot lysis. This enhanced ability to lyse clots appears to result primarily from an elevation of circulating plasminogen activator levels. Despite this rise, no fibrinogenolysis occurs, as evidenced by normal levels of fibrinogen and no elevation of fibrinogen degradation products during prolonged infusion of activated Protein C. This suggests that the role of the enzyme in clot lysis is different from those of urokinase or streptokinase, which activate circulating plasminogen to plasmin, with subsequent proteolysis of fibrinogen. Perfusion of isolated dog tissues does not release plasminogen activator from the vasculature. However, when activated Protein C is added to blood in vitro and subsequently neutralized with specific antibodies, the rate of clot lysis is increased when this blood is then reinjected into the animal. The addition of activated Protein C to plasma alone is sufficient to generate the fibrinolytic activity, but the effect is more marked when the enzyme is added to a mixture of plasma and blood cells. Comp and Esmon (16) have suggested that activated Protein C might generate a secondary messenger, which in turn causes the increase in circulating plasminogen activator activity.

Canfield and Kiesel (17) have recently succeeded in purifying to homogeneity an activated Protein C-binding protein from normal human plasma. This binding protein (mol. wt. 54,000) is a glycoprotein and possesses an amino-terminal sequence with considerable homology with bovine cholostrum inhibitor and pancreatic trypsin inhibitor, but no apparent sequence homology with the known plasma serine protease inhibitors. Affinity-purified antibody against this binding protein immunoprecipitated a complex of radiolabeled and native binding proteins from normal human plasma. There was essentially no complex formation in plasma immunodepleted of the binding protein. Thus,Protein C has an important physiological function in hemostasis, modulating clot formation and clot lysis. The effects of the enzyme are regulated, in turn, by a naturally-occurring inhibitor.

Clinical significance

The physiological role of Protein C is now less obscure and its clinical importance is becoming increasingly evident. Marlar and Griffin in 1980 (18) reported that Protein C inhibitory activity was detectable in plasma. This inhibitory activity could not be seen in plasmas from four unrelated patients with combined Factor V/VIII deficiency, but it was present in normal amounts in patients with isolated Factor V or Factor VIII deficiencies. Since activated Protein C readily destroys Factor V and Factor VIII coagulant activities (13), they suggested that the molecular basis for combined Factor V/VIII deficiency is the congenital lack of this inhibitor. Canfield and Kisiel (17) have recently confirmed that normal human plasma contains an inhibitor directed against activated Protein C. However, at variance with the findings of Marlar and Griffin, they found that plasma from four patients with combined Factor V/VIII deficiency inhibited the anticoagulant and amidolytic activities of activated human Protein C at essentially the same rate as normal pooled plasma. Furthermore, incubation of radio-labelled activated Protein C with either normal or combined factor V/VIII-deficient plasma resulted in complex formation at the same rate and to the same extent. Finally, quantitative electroimmunoassay indicated equal levels of activated Protein C binding protein in normal plasma and in plasma from the four patients with combined factor V/VIII deficiency. Therefore, the role of activated Protein C and its naturally occurring inhibitor in the pathophysiology of combined Factor V/VIII deficiency is still unsettled.

Since Protein C is a potent anticoagulant and profibrinolytic agent, one could hypothesize that an inherited deficiency of Protein C would cause a thrombophilic state. In 1981, Griffin et al (19) reported a family with a history of recurrent venous thromboembolism due to an inherited deficiency of Protein C. The propositus, his father and his paternal uncle had 38-49% of normal levels of Protein C antigen, whereas unaffected family members had normal levels. Since no assay of functional Protein C in plasma was available, the study of Protein C was limited to immunological assay. In 1982, Bertina et al (20) described a similar Dutch family with a history of thrombotic disease associated with an isolated deficiency of Protein C antigen.

In 1982 Mannucci and Viganò (21) reported data about acquired defects of Protein C. In healthy controls there were no differences in Protein C related to age or sex. The low levels found in 12 healthy full-term newborn infants are probably a reflection of liver immaturity at birth, also expressed in the low levels of vitamin K-dependent and contact - phase clotting factors. The Protein C levels in 20 women in the last trimester of normal pregnancy were no different from those in healthy non-pregnant women. Protein C concentrations were low in chronic liver disease, in degrees roughly proportional to the severity of the disease and thus to the impairment of protein synthesis, suggesting that the liver is probably the site of synthesis of this protein. However, one cannot rule out the possibility that low plasma concentrations of Protein C are due to increased turnover, as has previously been found for other haemostatic components in chronic liver disease.

In clinical conditions associated with disseminated intravascular coagulation (DIC), Protein C levels were very low and sometimes unmeasurable (21), the most likely explanation of this being that Protein C activated by thrombin during DIC is rapidly cleared from the circulation. It is possible that during DIC, anoxia or endotoxin (or both) could damage endothelial cells allowing the endothelial-cell cofactor to be exposed in greater than normal quantities; hence, Protein C activation would be much increased and its clearance from plasma accelerated. This hypothesis is supported by the finding of very low or unmeasurable levels of Protein C in adult respiratory distress syndrome, a condition characterized by extensive pulmonary endothelial damage. The period immediately after minor or major surgical operation was also associated with an acquired defect of Protein C (21). A possible explanation is that during surgery and immediately afterwards tissue damage induces an _in vivo_ activation of blood clotting, resulting in increased thrombin formation. In conjunction with the endothelial-cell cofactor, thrombin might in turn activate Protein C, leading to faster removal of Protein C from the circulation. Studies are currently in progress in our laboratory to ascertain the behaviour of Protein C in other acquired conditions, such as ischemic cerebrovascular disease, acute leukemias, intake of oral contraceptives, ischemic heart disease etc.

In conclusion, the recent availability of a simple and reproducible electroimmunoassay for Protein C antigen has allowed a considerable amount of information about the pathological role of this new vitamin K-dependent protein to be obtained. However the lack of a similarly reliable biological assay hampers drawing firm conclusions.

REFERENCES

1. Stenflo J. A new vitamin K-dependent protein. J.Biol.Chem 251: 355-63, 1976
2. Kisiel W. Human plasma protein C. J.Clin.Invest. 64:761-69,1979
3. Comp P.C., Jacobs R.M., Ferrell G.L. and Esmon C.T. Activation of protein C in vivo. J.Clin.Invest. 70: 127-34, 1982
4. Owen W., Esmon C.T. Functional properties of an endothelial cell cofactor for thrombin-catalyzed activation of protein C. J.Biol. Chem. 256: 5532-35, 1981
5. Esmon C.T., Owen W.G. Identification of an endothelial cell cofactor for thrombin-catalyzed activation of protein C. Proc.Natl.Acad.Sci. USA 78: 2249-52, 1981
6. Esmon N.L., Owen W.G. and Esmon C.T. Isolation of a membrane bound cofactor for thrombin catalyzed activation of protein C. J.Biol. Chem. 257: 859-64, 1982
7. Mammen E., Thomas W. and Seegers W.H. Activation of purified prothrombin to autoprothrombin I or autoprothrombin II (platelet cofactor II) or autoprothrombin II A. Thromb.Diath.Haemorrh.5, 218-250, 1960
8. Marciniak E. Inhibitor of human blood coagulation elicited by thrombin. J.Lab.Clin.Med. 79: 924-34, 1972
9. Murano G., Seegers W.H., Zolton R. Autoprothrombin IIA: a competitive inhibitor of autoprothrombin C. A review with additions. Throm.Haemorrh.Diath. (Suppl.) 57: 305-14, 1974
10. Seegers W.H., Marlar R.A., Wall D. Anticoagulant effects of autoprothrombin IIA and prothrombin fragment 1. Thromb.Res. 13: 233-43 1978
11. Esmon C., Comp P. and Walker F. Functions for protein C. In"vitamin K Metabolism and vitamin K-Dependent Proteins". J.Suttie Ed.:72-83 1980 University Park Press Baltimore, MD
12. Vehar G. and Davie E. Preparation and properties of bovine factor VIII (Antihemophilic factor) Biochemistry 19: 401-410, 1980
13. Marlar R.A., Kleiss A.J. and Griffin H.J. Mechanism of action of human activated protein C, a thrombin-dependent anticoagulant enzyme. Blood 59: 1067-72, 1982
14. Seegers W.H., McCoy C., Groben H., Sakuragawa N.,Agrawal B. Purification and some properties of autoprothrombin IIA: an anticoagulant perhaps related to fibrinolysis. Thromb.Res.1:443-60 19872
15. Zolton R.P. and Seegers W.H. Autoprothrombin IIA:thrombin removal and mechanism of induction of fibrinolysis. Thromb.Res.3:23-33 1973

16. Comp P.C. and Esmon C.T. Generation of fibrinolytic activity by infusion of activated protein C into dogs. J.Clin.Invest. 68:1221-28 1981
17. Canfield W.N. and Kiesel W. Evidence of normal functional levels of activated protein C inhibitor in combined factor V/VIII deficiency disease J.Clin.Invest. 70:1260-1272, 1982
18. Marlar R.A. and Griffin J.H. Deficiency of protein C inhibitor in combined factor V/VIII deficiency disease. J.Clin.Invest. 66: 1186-89,1980
19. Griffin J.H., Evatt B., Zimmerman T.S., Kiesel A.J. and Wideman C. Deficiency of protein C in congenital thrombotic disease. J.Clin.Invest. 68: 1370-73, 1981
20. Bertina R.M., Broekmans A.W., Van der Linden I.K. and Nerkens K. Protein C deficiency in a Dutch family with thrombotic disease. Thrombos.Haemostas 48 (1): 1-5, 1982
21. Mannucci P.M., Viganò S. Deficiencies of protein C, an inhibitor of blood coagulation. Lancet, 2: 463-467, 1982

DISCUSSION LECTURE MANNUCCI

Samama Why didn't you study the correlation between Protein C deficiency and pre-albumin, wich has a short half-life which we found useful in this kind of study?

Mannucci We did'nt, simply because this test pre-albumin is not used now in our liver unit as a routine test, we want to compare with a more routinary test, but I agree with you that you might provide certainly better correlation than with albumin, at least what one would expect.

Giddings Would you like to comment on the apparent paradoxical effect that you have when you administer warfarin in something you say clotting methods, and also administer protein C which is potentially antithrombotic?

Mannucci I think, I didn't mention it here because I simply want use that slide to give you an idea of the half-life of Protein C, but certainly it is very important that you a decrease of an inhibitor that gives a thrombotic tend at the time, when only Factor VII, which has not got an antithrombotic capacity, is decreased, and this might b of the reasons, probably not the only one, why in the e state of anticoagulant treatment, it has been shown tha there is no or very little antithrombotic action. There are all data suggesting this is so, and this is maybe a other reason why it is so and this reinforced the conce that heparin and oral anticoagulants should be overlapp for a longer period of time than it is usually done. I would say that seven days are the minimum. I do not certainly see the potency of Protein C in the time when only Factor VII is significant decrease might have a significance.

Verstraete You did mention a number of circumstances where you did find any change of Protein C. I wonder if you did also whether under anticontraceptive pill or the oral antico tives, because Factor VII does change and found some re tionship in both?

Mannucci We are doing it now with Prof. Mead in London, but we haven't yet done and yet obtained the results.

Verstraete Do you have any speculation on the continuously counter wich, deprived from the early phase of Coumarine therapy and could you explain if it has something to do with a drop of Factor VII?

Mannucci That is an interesting suggestion, I don't know but it's a very interesting idea.

Question from the audience

Mannucci I cannot answer, the only thing I can tell you is that in our group, in our hands as much as there was a proportional decrease of Protein C in the progressive forms, I mean more in chronic active and chronic persistance and more in cirrhosis than in chronic active this was also true for other indexes of liver synthetic capacity, that is albumin, choline-esterase and prothrombin time. So, in our hands, in our patients, we found that even patients with chronic active hepatitis had less decrease of protein synthesis than patients with cirrhosis or like what you seem to have suggested. I think it might depend on the type of patients. I don't know whether this gives you any hint. Our patients were usually not alcoholic and you know that in our countries the spectrum of liver disease in Italy is somewhat different that it is in countries from Northern Europe. I am internist and not a specialist hepatologist.
But in our department they use some expertising days and this may be what my colleague says. In any way it would be interesting to look at the appearance of the histological part and to evaluate what you have suggested.

INTRAVASCULAR COAGULATION IN LIVER DISEASE

D. COLLEN

INTRODUCTION

Severe liver disease is frequently associated with a bleeding tendency and/or abnormalities in the laboratory tests of hemostasis. The latter comprise deficiencies of one or more of the coagulation factors II, V, VII, IX, X, XI, and XIII, thrombocytopenia and/or thrombocytopathia, and increased fibrinolytic activity in the plasma.

Several mechanisms are thought to be involved in the pathogenesis of these disturbances. The decreased levels of coagulation factors have generally been ascribed to impaired hepatic synthesis. An increased consumption of coagulation factors due to intravascular coagulation has been proposed as an alternative or complementary cause of the depletion of coagulation factors.

The fibrinolytic response to stimuli such as injection of nicotinic acid in cirrhosis of the liver is exagerated. It was therefore suggested that abnormal fibrinolysis in the cirrhotic patient may be due to a failure of the hepatic clearance of plasminogen activator. The exagerated fibrinolytic response in cirrhosis may be facilitated by decreased levels of circulating inhibitors. Serum α_2-antiplasmin levels were found to be reduced in patients with liver insufficiency.

TURNOVER OF FIBRINOGEN, PROTHROMBIN, AND PLASMINOGEN IN LIVER DISEASE

Measurement of the turnover rate of radiolabeled components of the coagulation and fibrinolytic systems allows a quantitative determination of the relative importance of defective synthesis, intravascular coagulation, and fibrinolysis in the pathogenesis of the coagulation disturbances in liver disease. A decrease in the level of circulating fibrinogen, prothrombin, and plasminogen will only occur when the synthesis is markedly impaired or when the rate of catabolism is so excessively enhanced that maximal synthesis fails to compensate. Therefore, turnover studies of these factors could be particularly useful to study the kinetics of synthesis and breakdown and to differentiate their catabolic pathways in states of altered coagulability.

Tytgat et al. (1) studied the metabolism of homologous human fibrinogen labeled with radioactive iodine in 50 patients with well documented cirrhosis of the liver. These patients were at various stages of the disease, but in a steady state with respect to fibrinogen metabolism. The mean plasma fibrinogen concentration of 250 mg $\pm$ 102 mg/100 ml in cirrhosis was not significantly lower than the control value of 284 $\pm$ 71 mg/100 ml in thirty five control subjects. The mean fibrinogen half-life of 2.99 $\pm$ 0.59 days was significantly shorter than the half-life of 4.14 $\pm$ 0.56 days in controls, whereas the mean fractional catabolic rate of 0.34 $\pm$ 0.09 of the plasma pool/day in cirrhosis was significantly higher than the control value of 0.24 $\pm$ 0.04. The mean quantity of fibrinogen catabolized daily, 2.66 $\pm$ 1.43 g or 39 $\pm$ 20 mg/kg in cirrhotics, was significantly higher than the corresponding mean control values of 1.94 $\pm$ 0.59 g or 28 $\pm$ 9 mg/kg. On the average the increased fibrinogen catabolism was counterbalanced by increased synthesis resulting in normal plasma fibrinogen levels.

During continuous heparin infusion in 10 cirrhotic patients the fibrinogen half-life was prolonged from 3.15 $\pm$ 0.69 to 4.59 $\pm$ 0.79 days. Inhibition of the fibrinolytic system by peroral administration of tranexamic acid did not influence the fibrinogen half-life consistently. It was therefore concluded that the accelerated fibrinogen consumption was mainly due to continuous intravascular coagulation.

The plasma levels of prothrombin, the zymogen which is finally converted in the coagulation mechanism, and of plasminogen, the precursor of the fibrinolytic enzyme plasmin, are frequently subnormal in cirrhosis of the liver. This may be the result of either diminished hepatic synthesis, or excessive consumption, or both.

Turnover studies of labeled prothrombin, prepared by the method of Swart (2), have been performed by Collen et al. (3) in six patients with cirrhosis of the liver to evaluate the relative importance of defective synthesis and in vivo coagulation in the pathogenesis of the hypoprothrombinemia. Compared to normals, the cirrhotic patients showed a significantly increased fractional catabolic rate and a decreased synthetic rate. Heparin administration in three patients resulted in a normalization of the prothrombin half-life. However, because the plasma prothrombin level was correlated with the synthetic rate but not with the fractional catabolic rate, it was concluded that the hypoprothrombinemia was mainly caused by the impaired synthetic ability of the diseased liver.

Turnover studies of labeled plasminogen (3), performed in four patients with cirrhosis of the liver, revealed an increased fractional catabolic rate and a decreased synthesis rate of plasminogen; heparin administration in two patients resulted in a normalization of the turnover rate. As was observed for prothrombin, the plasma plasminogen level was correlated with the synthetic rate but not with the fractional catabolic rate, indicating that the hypoplasminogenemia was also mainly the result of decreased synthesis.

Two hypotheses can be presented to explain the accelerated plasminogen catabolism in cirrhosis : primary or secondary activation of the fibrinolytic system or absorption of plasminogen onto in vivo evolving fibrin. The absence of overt signs of fibrinolytic activity does not necessarily invalidate the hypothesis of primary or secondary activation of the fibrinolytic system. Indeed the dynamic study of the plasminogen turnover should be much more sensitive in detecting accelerated consumption than the static picture of circulating levels of plasminogen, plasminogen activator, or fibrin(ogen) degradation products.

PATHOGENESIS OF INTRAVASCULAR COAGULATION IN SEVERE LIVER DISORDERS

A reasonable explanation for the occurrence of intravascular coagulation in patients with severe liver insufficiency is that necrotic hepatocytes are the initial trigger. In addition, activated coagulation factors are less opposed because of defective clearing in the reticuloendothelial system and lowered levels of antithrombin in liver disease. These different elements are now analyzed in some detail.

Consumption coagulopathy is often seen in states where blood comes into contact with damaged cells; tissue thromboplastin-like material is released in response to cellular injury, with consequent activation of the coagulation process and thrombin-induced aggregation of platelets. The original stimulus to intravascular coagulation in liver disease probably comes from the necrotic hepatocytes. The clearance of procoagulants thus generated may be diminished because of liver insufficiency (4). Furthermore, in cirrhotic patients the expanded collateral circulation and congested spleen represent a tremendous increase in endothelial surface. Sluggish circulation in this collateral vascular bed and in dilated splenic sinusoids, where a high number of platelets are trapped, might well create (hypoxic?) alterations of the endothelial cells and predispose to local clotting. This hypothesis is supported by the finding of a shortened fibrinogen half-life in patients with extrahepatic portal hypertension, splenomegaly, and extensive collateral circulation but with normal liver function and architecture (1). Some similarity can be seen between the extensive collateral circulation in cirrhosis and a giant hemangioma, which is also frequently associated with intravascular coagulation (5,6). As overt hemolysis of different degrees is often a feature in liver cirrhosis (7), release of phospholipid and adenosine diphosphate from the red cells could also trigger in vivo coagulation and platelet aggregation. Thus in patients with severe liver insufficiency a variety of stimuli for the initiation of in vivo coagulation is present.

Since intravascular fibrin thrombi in the liver sinusoids were observed in toxic hepatic necrosis (8) and can cause further liver damage, and since fragmentation of red cells (so-called microangiopathic hemolytic anemia) may cause further release of thromboplastic material, a vicious circle may result which can perpetuate intravascular coagulation.

Activated coagulation factors are normally rapidly removed from the blood stream due to the clearing function of the liver. This property was convincingly demonstrated in animals by Wessler et al. (4) and Deykin (9). When thrombin-free normal human serum was injected through the marginal vein of a rabbit, a hypercoagulable state was produced, resulting in rapid clot formation in an isolated venous segment (4). The infusion of thrombin-free normal human serum through the portal vein accelerated the rate of attenuation of the hypercoagulable response. In contrast, occlusion of the hepatic circulation after the injection of serum prolonged the hypercoagulable state, and widespread thrombosis occurred in areas of vascular stasis. Finally it was shown that the thrombogenic activity of normal human serum was cleared by perfusion through isolated rabbit liver (9). Furthermore, the liver possesses a remarkable capacity to distinguish between the nonactivated and activated clotting factors, only the latter being very efficiently removed from the bloodstream (10).

When minute amounts of thrombin are generated, the action of this enzyme can also more readily develop when the antithrombin level is reduced, as is often observed in patients with liver insufficiency.

CONCLUSION

It can be concluded that the biological integrity of the liver cell system appears of utmost importance in preventing in vivo activation of the coagulation system. Not only are the liver cells the principal site of synthesis of the bulk of coagulation and fibrinolytic proteins, but they are also invaluable in equilibrating clot-promoting forces.

It is presently well documented that the levels of certain coagulation factors are decreased in severe liver insufficiency. Furthermore, the catabolism of fibrinogen, prothrombin and plasminogen is enhanced in liver cirrhosis. The consistent normalization of the fibrinogen half-life by heparin administration strongly suggests that continuous low-grade in vivo coagulation is responsible for the increased catabolism; usually the increased metabolism is counterbalanced by an enhanced synthesis resulting in normal plasma fibrinogen levels. On the contrary, the decreased levels of prothrombin and plasminogen frequently encountered in this condition are mainly due to an insufficient synthesis and only to a minor degree to enhanced catabolism.

Although the present data indicate that low-grade intravascular coagulation is a frequent complication of severe liver disease, overt consumption coagulopathies requiring therapeutic anticoagulation are rare.

REFERENCES

1. Tytgat GN, Collen D, Verstraete M. 1971. Metabolism of fibrinogen in cirrhosis of the liver. J.Clin.Invest. 50, 1690-1701.
2. Swart ACW. 1971. Studies on the purification and separation of blood coagulation factors II, VII, IX and X. Ph.D.-thesis, University of Leiden.
3. Collen D, Rouvier J, Chamone DF, Verstraete M. 1978. Turnover of radiolabelled plasminogen and prothrombin in cirrhosis of the liver. Eur.J. Clin.Invest. 8, 185-199.
4. Wessler S, Yin ET, Gaston LW, Nicol I. 1967. A distinction between the role of precursor and activated forms of clotting factors in the genesis of stasis thrombi. Thromb.Diath.haemorrh. 18, 12-23.
5. Verstraete M, Vermylen C, Vermylen J, Vandenbroucke J. 1965. Excessive consumption of blood coagulation components as cause of hemorrhagic diathesis. Amer.J.Med. 38, 899-908.
6. Blix S, Aas K. 1961. Giant haemangioma, thrombocytopenia, fibrinogenopenia, and fibrinolytic activity. Acta Med.Scand. 169, 63-70.
7. Kimber CJ, Deller DJ, Ibbotson RN, Lander H. 1965. The mechanism of anaemia in chronic liver disease. Quart.J.Med. 34, 33-64.
8. Popper H, Franklin M. 1948. Viral versus toxic hepatic necrosis. Arch. Pathol. 46, 338-376.
9. Deykin D. 1966. The role of the liver in serum-induced hypercoagulability. J.Clin.Invest. 45, 256-263.
10. Deykin D, Cochios F, Decamp G, Lopez A. 1968. Hepatic removal of activated factor X by the perfused rabbit liver. Am.J.Physiol. 214, 414-419.

DISCUSSION LECTURE COLLEN

Vinazzer I have one question about the heparin test.
In these cases when production of clotting factor is low, production of antithrombin III is also low, and if you have a low antithrombin III, the heparin cannot act on coagulation. Would you comment on this?

Collen Well, this is a problem that apparently has been discussed and debated on many occasions. If you look at the affinity between heparin and antithrombin III, the dissociation constant that is very well determined, than it appears that in a patient with a normal antithrombin III level, when you inject a bolus of 5000 units, actually most of it will go to the antithrombin III, and that when the level of antithrombin III decreases to 30 percent, which may occur in some of these patients, but that already seldom rarily below this, that you will still have an anticoagulant efficiency of your heparin, which is at least 1/3 of that in normals. So, really, I think that before a patient becomes refractory to heparin, that the levels have to be so low to a level that you rarely encounter in liver disease. That is my believe.

Samama I think I may add that in a purified system,unless antithrombin III is lower than 50%, you have no difference in the effect of heparin as in antithrombin III purified system. Do you agree, Dr. Vinazzer, that in a purified system with antithrombin III 50-100% the activity of heparin is not modified?

Vinazzer In purified system O.K. But in patients, AT III level lower than 50% gives thrombotic tendency.

Question from the audience

Collen Yes, it is evident that the efficiency of heparin-anticoagulation will be inversely proportional to the level of antithrombin III; if you have a higher antithrombin III level, you will form more 'heparin-antithrombin III-complex' but really the level has to decrease very significantly before the patient becomes refractory to heparin. So in

these cases of continuous low grade intravascular coagul tion the amount of circulating heparin-antithrombin III complexes that you need to counter-balance this is a tra amount really.
The acceleration of the inhibition of antithrombin III following complex formation with heparin is about 2000-f so what you need in order to double the anticoagulation potential of antithrombin III by making heparin-antithro III complexes is to convert 1/10 of a percent of the cir ting antithrombin III into heparin-antithrombin III comp Then you double it. Of course if you want to increase th anticoagulant level by a factor 10 or 100, then it is ev that you need significant steady-state concentrations in blood of heparin-antithrombin III complex, but apparently counterbalance these low-grade intravascular coagulation the amount of anticoagulation you have to do is extremel low, and this is also confirmed by the low-grade heparin anticoagulation that is apparently performed in the post-operative phase. The levels of circulating heparin-antithrombin III that you need in order to have an antithrombotic effect appears to be very low, so low that most coagulation assays cannot detect. This level of anticoagular you need this specific very sensitive Factor Xa inhibitic assay for that.

Brommer (Question)

Collen Well, there is some information in patients. I can rememb 2 studies that are almost 15 years old, where nicotinic a injection were performed in normals and in patients with disease. In normals, nicotinic acid will increase the cir ting level of plasminogen activator by a factor 3 on aver The half-life of that plasminogen activator activity in t blood is 13 minutes from the study of Tytgat. In liver-ci sis, the half-life will be about 14 minutes. That is one thing. The other thing is that we have studied the tu over of labeled tissue plasminogen activator in rabbits a measured where the iodine goes. It goes very quickly to t liver and if you do the surgical hepatectomy, or function hepatectomy by tying off the liver vessels, than the life-time becomes very long. So, I believe that it is really going to the liver. It is broken down there rapidly.

Question from the audience

Collen Yes, well, apparently you deplete the stores of plasminogen activator very abruptly, very easily. So I think that although that value of 13 minutes may be somewhat longer than the real half-life it gives you some significant information of the clearance time in humans, which is than supported by animal work where it is in my view clearly proved. Labeled plasminogen activator goes to the liver.

ABNORMALITIES OF FIBRIN FORMATION IN SEVERE HEPATIC DISEASES.

J. SORIA, C. SORIA - Service des Professeurs Bernadou-Fabiani-Samama

Bleeding is a common complication in severe hepatic diseases. The mechanism of bleeding is complex and many causes are involved such as :

- Decrease in blood coagulation factors which are synthetized in the liver.
- Thrombocytopenia and platelet dysfunctions.
- Acquired fibrinolysis and intravascular coagulation (DIC).
- Abnormal fibrin formation observed in severe acute or chronic hepatic failure. This finding is complex and requires a special investigation.

Table I summarizes some factors involved in the abnormality of fibrin formation.

Table I : Acquired fibrin formation abnormality in severe hepatic diseases

I. - Hypofibrinogenemia
2. - Abnormal fibrin polymerization with normal level of plasma fibrinogen :
- presence of plasma inhibitor,
- acquired dysfibrinogenemia.

I. HYPOFIBRINOGENEMIA IN SEVERE HEPATIC DISEASES.

Fibrinogen is synthetized in the liver. The measurement of plasma fibrinogen (8), however, is not a good index of liver function, as reported by Poller (28) : fibrinogen was only found to be depressed in the very severe cases of hepatic failure but the fibrinogen level was less affected than other specific clotting factors. Normal levels of fibrinogen were reported by several authors (II, 28, 42, 43) in patients with cirrhosis and portal hypertension.

Hypofibrinogenemia may be related to various causes such as :

1. Decreased synthesis.

Green et al (I7) showed that the decrease in the fibrinogen level is not useful in assessing the degree of hepatic liver dysfunction, because other clinical processes which occur in cirrhosis and hepatic obstruction, such as inflammatory lesions, induce an increase of fibrinogen synthesis (I7). Thus, the relationship of decreased fibrinogen level to the degree of liver dysfunction only appears to be close in the very severe cases.

2. Increased catabolic pathway.

This mechanism has been implicated in some cases of hypofibrinogenemia. Tytgat (43) and Rake (3I) have shown that the mean half life of fibrinogen is decreased in cirrhosis but usually this increased rate of catabolism is counterbalanced by an increased synthesis.

- The role of fibrinolysis in the haemostatic defect of liver failure was reviewed by Collen.
- Disseminated intravascular coagulation (DIC) (3,45). A decrease of fibrinogen level in plasma may possibly be due to DIC. The causes of DIC in liver disease are important, such as :
  - deficiency in the liver clearance of activated clotting factors.
  - tissue necrosis inducing activation of blood coagulation.
  - reduction of inhibitors of blood coagulation (such as AT III and protein C clearly shown by Manucci, predisposing to DIC (24).

Nevertheless, the diagnosis of DIC is quite difficult to prove. Tytgat et al in I97I (43) and Coleman et al in I975 (9) showed that heparin prolonged the half life of labelled fibrinogen in the cirrhotic patient. Although classical laboratory tests gave no convincing data to support DIC in severe cirrhosis, ethanol gelation test is usually negative, and the level of FDP in serum is in the upper limit range. We have found, however, that the detection of soluble complexes in plasma using the haemagglutination test described by Largo et al (2I) gave much better results and it appeared at least seven fold more times sensitive than the ethanol gelation test (40). This test consists of the haemagglutination of red blood cells sensitized with fibrin monomers by fibrin monomers from patient's plasma, as seen in fig. 1

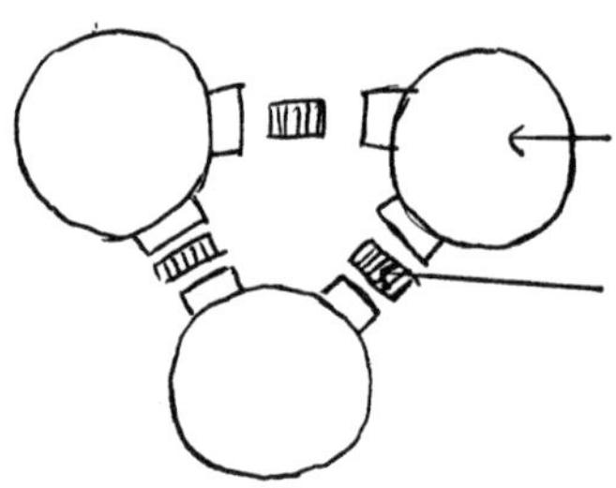

Fig. 1 : Haemagglutination test for detection of fibrin monomers in plasma.

We have shown that the haemagglutination test is positive in 30 % of patients with cirrhosis, having a level of fibrinogen less than 200 mg/I00 ml. Coccheri and other authors (I0, 29) using the detection of high molecular weight fibrin derivatives by gel filtration and the determination of fibrinopeptide A (fpA) level in plasma, have reached the same conclusion. Because the haemagglutination test of Largo is very easy to perform, we suggest including this test, in order to dedect DIC in patients suffering from cirrhosis. Furthermore, unlike the ethanol gelation test, this assay is not influenced by the level of fibrinogen and therefore no false negatives were observed in cases of DIC with low levels of fibrinogen (40).

II ABNORMAL FIBRIN POLYMERIZATION

Fibrin formation evaluation by the thrombin and reptilase clotting times, is abnormal in some cases of severe liver disease. Three mechanisms may be implicated for the abnormal fibrin formation as shown in table II.

Table II : Abnormal fibrin formation in severe liver disease.

Prolongation of the thrombin clotting time

- Acquired dysfibrinogenemia
- Partial degradation of the Aα chain of fibrinogen.
- Presence of an inhibitor of fibrin formation

Anomaly was detected both in plasma and in isolated fibrinogen. (Acquired dysfibrinogenemia; partial degradation of the Aα chain)

Abnormality of fibrinoformation was absent using purified fibrinogen. (Presence of an inhibitor)

Abnormal fibrinogen can be confirmed if the anomaly is found in both plasma and purified fibrinogen. But abnormal fibrin polymerization may be also due to the existence of a plasma inhibitor. In this last case, thrombin and reptilase clotting times are prolonged when plasma is tested, whereas they are normal with isolated fibrinogen samples (28, 39).

A) Abnormal fibrinogen in liver disease.

In the present classification, the qualitative fibrinogen abnormality is divided into 2 groups :

- In the first, the functional defect is due to an acquired dysfibrinogenemia,
- In the second, the anomaly is related to a partial degradation of fibrinogen by proteolytic enzymes.

1. Acquired dysfibrinogenemia

The first case of acquired dysfibrinogenemia was observed in I968 in our laboratory (37) in a case of severe hepatitis. We the looked for this anomaly and found it in some cases (38, 39) :

- 4 patients had severe viral hepatitis. The anomaly disappeared when the patient recovered.
- 5 patients were observed among I83 cases of liver cirrhosis.
- In 2 cases, the acquired dysfibrinogenemia was associated with a primary hepatoma, as were the cases reported by Von Felten et al (46) and Verhaeghe (44), and the case of Gralnick (I6). In 2 other cases of hepatoma, fibrinogen was qualitatively normal.
- The anomaly was also detected in toxic hepatitis, as was shown by Poller and coworkers (30). Green et al (I7) Martinez (25, 26), Francis (I3), Coccheri (IO), Gralnick (I6), Lane (20) and Palaretti (28) have also found acquired dysfibrinogenemia in hepatic disease.

Diagnosis of dysfibrinogenemia :

The abnormality is discovered because of a prolonged thrombin and reptilase clotting times. The kinetic variation of optical density (OD) induced by addition of thrombin (or reptilase) to diluted plasma (or fibrinogen) allows the global exploration of the 2 first phases of fibrin formation (4) ; 2 types of curves can be observed (fig. 2) :

- a flat curve showing coagulation with no modification of OD (Translucent clot).
- elongated curve with a maximum OD corresponding to the level of fibrinogen indicating a delayed fibrin polymerization.

The first eventuality is the most frequent.

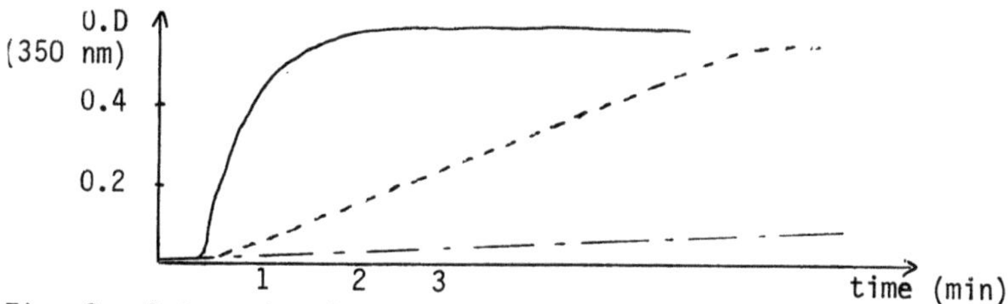

Fig. 2 : Polymerization curve of fibrin formation after addition of thrombin to normal plasma (—) or patient plasma (---- and—·—), diluted in 0.15 M NaCl in order to obtain 30 mg/100 ml fibrinogen (final concentration).

The decrease of the ionic strength of the diluting buffer attenuate the abnormality, (this seems to be explained by the fact that hydrogen bonds are formed more easily when the ionic strength is decreased).

The presence of qualitative disorder of fibrinogen can only be confirmed in these patients if the anomaly is found in purified fibrinogen : after isolation of fibrinogen by the Blombäck procedure (2), both the thrombin time and the spectrophotometric study of fibrin formation are abnormal.

In such cases, the defect of fibrinogen is not related to a degradation of the molecule as shown by polyacrylamide gel electrophoresis, performed in the presence of SDS (PAGE-SDS) of the 3 chains of fibrinogen previously dissociated by urea and mercaptoethanol (34) : the molecular weight of the 3 chains are similar in normal and patient's fibrinogen (fig. 3).

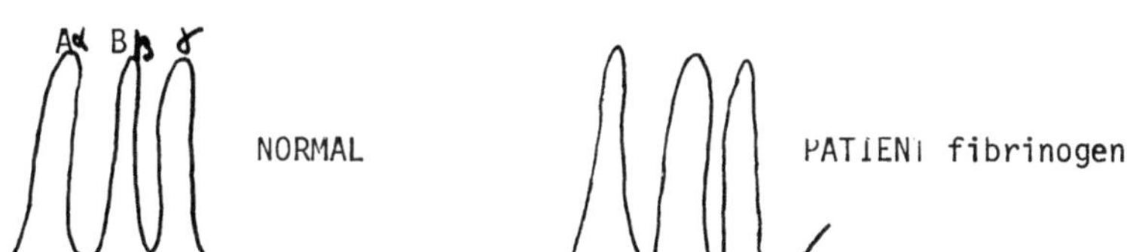

Fig. 3 : Polyacrylamide gel electrophoresis in the presence of SDS of normal fibrinogen and fibrinogen from acquired dysfibrinogenemia in hepatic disease.

Analysis of the 3 stages of fibrin formation.

- Kinetic release of fpA and fpB : thrombin was added to purified fibrinogen. Three assays were performed :
  1. After separation of fibrinopeptides from fibrinogen by bentonite adsorption, fpA determination was performed by an immunoenzymological procedure (4I).
  2. Fibrinopeptides released from fibrinogen were separated from fibrinogen, fibrin monomers and fibrin according to their molecular weight (we used the solutibity of fibrinopeptides in trichloracetic acid) and the concentration of both fibrinopeptides A and B was determined by Lowry's procedure.
  3. Determination of fibrinopeptide release by HPLC procedure as described by Kehl et al (I8).

Using these assays, release of fibrinopeptides was normal in acquired dysfibrinogenemia.

- Aggregation of fibrin monomers (I)

Aggregation of fibrin monomers, previously isolated by dissociation of the hydrogen bonds in a non-stabilized clot, was studied by the continuous measurement of optical density when monomers were diluted in a buffer, allowing the formation of hydrogen bonds. The abnormality of fibrin formation in acquired dysfibrinogenemia, is related to an abnormal fibrin monomer polymerization. The increasing opacity due to the aggregation of fibrin monomers is absent in most cases and sometimes delayed.

- Stabilization of fibrin by activated factor XIII :

The formation by transamidase linkages induced by activated factor XIII between 2 γ chains of 2 different monomers and several α chains of different monomers, were studied by SDS-polyacrylamide gel electrophoresis (34). The formation of γ dimers and α polymers was normal in stabilized fibrin from patients having acquired dysfibrinogenemia.

- Study of the fibrinogen molecule

Abnormalities of the carbohydrate fractions have been

noticed in these abnormal fibrinogens. Sialic acid content measured by Warren procedure (47) was always elevated and there was a strong correlation between the thrombin clotting time, sialic acid content and content in purified fibrinogen as shown by Mester (27), by our group (33, 38, 39), by Palacaz and Martinez (29, 25, 26) and more recently by Francis (I3). The normal range of sialic acid is 6.2 ± 0.5 µg/mg of fibrinogen. In patients fibrinogen, the level of sialic acid increased up to I2 µg/mg of fibrinogen. The increase in sialic acid in the molecule of fibrinogen is responsible for the abnormality of fibrin formation, because the correction of sialic acid content by treatment with neuraminidase induces the normalization of fibrin formation (I3, 25, 26, 29, I4, 7) measured by thrombin clotting time and by the fibrin polymerization curves, as shown in fig. 4 and table II.

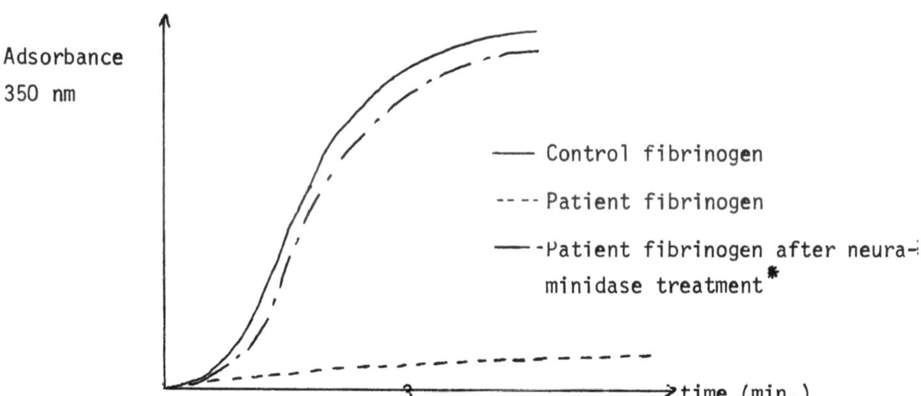

*Before treatment by neuraminidase, sialic and content was 10 µg/mg in patient fibrinogen.

After treatment by neuraminidase, sialic and content was 5 µg/mg in patient fibrinogen

Fig. 4 : Fibrin polymerization curve in control and patient fibrinogen before and after treatment by neuraminidase.

Fibrinogen tested	Content in Sialic Acid (µg/mg fibrinogen)	Thrombin time (sec.)
Control	0.55	24
Patient :		
- Before Neuraminidase Treatment	0.9	48
- After Neuraminidase Treatment	0.5	25

Table III : Relationship between sialic acid content in fibrinogen molecule and thrombin clotting time.

The incubation time of fibrinogen with Neuraminidase was carried out in order to normalize the level of sialic acid content. The reaction was stopped by gel filtration on sepharose 4B.

Furthermore, as shown by Green et al (17), in the presence of calcium, the abnormality of fibrin formation in acquired dysfibrinogenemia is less intense. We suggest that calcium may accelerate the fibrin formation also noted by Boyer (5). by neutralizing the negative charges of sialic acid.

The determination of the other carbohydrate in fibrinogen has been carried out: after hydrochloric acid hydrolysis, the carbohydrates were incorporated in a borate complex and then separated on a column on DA-X_8-11 using a liquimat II Kontron. The determination of each carbohydrate in the eluate was performed using Cu bis cinchoninate. The area of each peak was calculated. As shown in table IV, the content of galactose, mannose and N-acetyl-glucosamine was higher in patient's fibrinogen than in the normal one.

Carbohydrate in nmole/nmole of fibrinogen in :

	Control	Patients M...	W....	N....	M.....
N acetyl GLU	24	29	32	34	37
Mannose -	14	17	18	16	18
Galactose-	10	14	14	15	15

Table IV : Analysis of the carbohydrate moity of normal and patient's fibrinogen.

According to the work of Serafini-Cessi (35), the increase of sialic acid content in the fibrinogen molecule is due to an increased activity of sialyltransferase by regenerated cells. This hypothesis is supported by the facts that :

1° Sialyl -transferase is released in larger amounts by hepatoma cells, than normal hepatic cells,

2° An increase in sialyl transferase activity was found in serum from patients with hepatomas. Furthermore, the same increase in sialic acid content was also noted in other proteins such as in vitamin BI2-binding protein (6).

Increased activity of galactosyl-transferase could explain the high content of galactose in fibrinogen from acquired dysfibrinogenemia. But in contrast to sialyl-transferase, galactosyl-transferase in culture medium of hepatoma cells is comparable to that of normal hepatocytes (I9). Our results are in good agreement with those of Martinez, who showed that fibrinogen from patients with acquired dysfibrinogenemia, had a similar increase in sialic acid, galactose and mannose, which are associated with fibrinogen molecules through glycosyl-transferase in the external part of the glycosidic chains and a normal value of mannose, which is bound through the dolichol phosphate cycle, in the core, as seen in fig. 5.

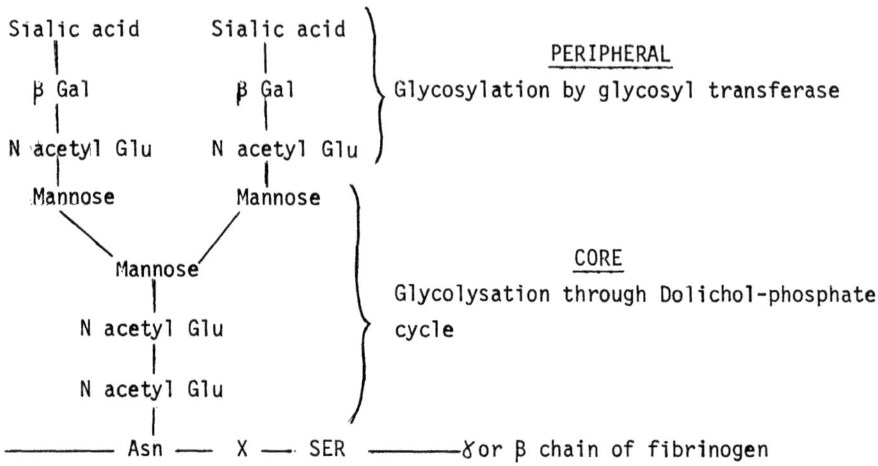

Fig. 5 : Carbohydrate moity of fibrinogen

In cirrhosis, acquired dysgibrinogenemia is only observed in severe hepatic disease and the presence of an abnormal fibrinogen indicates a poor prognosis. In severe viral hepatitis, acquired dysfibrinogenemia has been noted in the acute phase of the infection, and disappeared when the patient recovered. Therefore, the presence of dysfibrinogenemia cannot be taken into account for the prognosis in viral hepatitis. Furthermore, there was no bleeding complication that could be correlated with the abnormal fibrinogen.

2. Partial degradation of fibrinogen

This degradation in hepatic disease was described by Lipinski (22, 23) and was also noted by Weinstein and Deykin (48). In fact, this anomaly is seldomly encountered when fibrinogen is isolated in the presence of antifibrinolytic agent such as aprotinin. In our experiment, partial degradation of the A α chain was only found in one case out of I5 examined, as shown by SDS-PAGE (fig. 6) (only A α chain is degraded because it is very sensitive to proteolytic degradation).

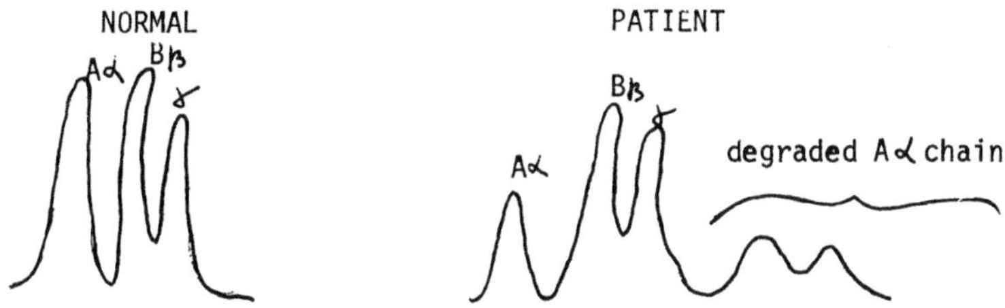

Fig. 6 : PAGE-SDS of the dissociated chains of fibrinogen

B) Presence of an inhibitor of fibrin formation

The presence of dysfibrinogenemia in patients with hepatic disease and prolonged thrombin clotting time can only be confirmed in these patients if the anomaly is found in purified fibrinogen. Thus, in 1974 (15) Gouault-Heilmann et al have shown that in a patient with liver disease, the abnormal polymerization was due to the existence of a plasmatic inhibitor and not to dysfibrinogenemia. In our study, (39) and in the study of Palaretti (28), the prolongation of thrombin and the presence of a translucent clot in some patients, is also explained by the presence of a plasmatic inhibitor, because the abnormality of fibrin polymerization was found in plasma and not found in isolated fibrinogen. In some of these cases, it is quite difficult to demonstrate an anticoagulant activity in serum, and we suggest that the inhibitor may circulate only in plasma because it is bound to fibrinogen.

CONCLUSION

In the past few years, there have been advances in our understanding of the abnormal fibrin formation acquired in hepatic disease. The occurence of DIC has been shown in advanced liver disease and has led to numerous reports and clinical trials which are not resolved. The presence of abnormal fibrinogen reflects severe hepatic disease, although it is however reversible in acute hepatitis such as viral hepatitis. The study of fibrinogen in cases of dysfibrinogenemia should bring useful information on the different functions of the molecule.

1. BELITSER, V.A., VARETSKAJA, T.V. and MALVENA, G.V. : Fibrinogen-fibrin interaction. Biochem. Biophys. Acta, 154, 367-372, 1968.

2. BLOMBACK, B., and BLOMBACK, M. Purification of human and bovine fibrinogen. Arkiv. Kemi., 10, 415-443, 1956.

3. BLOOM, A.L. Annotation. Intravascular coagulation and the liver. Brit. J. of Haematology, 30, 1, 1975.

4. BOUVIER, C. and GRUEDLINGER, J. Etude des phénomènes de coagulation et de fibrinolyse par une méthode simple d'enregistrement optique. Schweiz. Med. Wschr., 93, 1441-1443, 1963.

5. BOYER, R.D., SHAINOFF,J.R., RATNOFF, O.D. : Acceleration of fibrin polymerization by calcium ions. Blood, 39 : 382-387, 1972.

6. BURGER, R.L., WAXMAN, S., GILBERT, H.S., MEHLMAN, C.S., ALLEN, R.H. : Isolation and characterization of a novel vitamin B12-binding protein associated with hepatocellular carcinoma. J. Clin. Invest., 56, 1262-1270, 1975.

7. CHANDRASEKHAR, N., WARREN, L., OSBAHR, A.J., LAKI, K. : Role of sialic acid in fibrinogen. Biochim. Biophys. Acta, 63, 337-339, 1962.

8. CLAUSS, A. : Gerinnungsphysiologische schnellmethode zur bestimmung des fibrinogens. Acta Haemat., Basel, 17, 237-246, 1957.

9. COLEMAN, M., FINLAYSON, N., BETTIGOLE, R.E., SADULA, D., COHN, M. & PASMANTLER, M. : Fibrinogen survival in cirrhosis ; improvement by low dose hepatin. Annals of International Medicine, 83, 79, 1975.

10. COCCHERI, S., PALARETI, G., POGGI, M. : Fibrinogen in liver cirrhosis-fibrin monomer complexes and dysfibrinogenemia with high sialic acid content In "Fibrinogen recent advances and medical aspects (edited by A. HENSCHEN, H. GRAEFF, F. LOTTSPEICH, 329-337, 1982 (Walter de Gruyter).

11. DONALDSON, W.K., DAVIES, S.H., DARG, A. & RICHARDSON, J. : Coagulation factors in liver disease. Journal of Clinical Pathology, 22, 199,1969.

12. FELTON, A., VON STRAUB, P.W., FRICK, P.G. : Dysfibrinogenaemia in a patient with primary hepatoma. First observation of an acquired abnormality of fibrin monomer aggregation. New Engl. J. Med, 280, 405-409, 1969.

13. FRANCIS, J.L., ARMSTRONG, D.J. : Fibrinogen-bound sialic acid levels in the dysfibrinogenemia of liver diseases. Haemostasis, 11, 215-222, 1982.

14. GALANAKIS, D.K., MOSESSON, M.W. : Correction of the delayed fibrin aggregation of fetal fibrinogen by partial removal of sialic acid. VIIth Int. Congr. Thromb. Haemostasis. Abstract n° 0183, p. 79, 1979.

15. GOUAULT-HEILMANN, M., CHARDON, E., YVART, J., SULTAN, C. & CATTAN, D. Un cas d'hypofibrinogénémie congénitale avec trouble de la polymérisation de la fibrine au cours d'une cirrhose hépatique. Pathologie et Biologie, suppl. 21, 80, 1974.

16. GRALNICK, H.R., GIVELBER, H., and ABRAMS, E. : Dysfibrinogenaemia associated with hepatoma. Increased carbohydrate content of the fibrinogen molecule. New Engl. J. Med., 229, 221-226, 1978.

17. GREEN, G., THOMPSON, J.M., DYMOCK, I.M., POLLER L. : Abnormal fibrin polymerization in liver discase. Br. J. Haemat., 34, 425-439, 1976.

18. KEHL, M., LOTTSPEICH, F., HENSCHEN, A. : Analysis of human fibrinopeptides. by high performance liquid chromatography : quantitative determination and kinetics of release. In "Fibrinogen. Recent Biochemical and Medical Aspects. Editors (A. HENSCHEN, H. GRAEFF, F. LOTTSPEICH). Walter de GRUYTER, p 217-228, 1982.

19. KIM, Y.S. , PERDOMO, J., WHITEHEAD, J.S., CURTIS K.J. : glycosyltransferase in human blood. Study of serum galactosyltransferase and N-acetyl galactosaminyltransferase in patients with liver diseases. J. Clin. Invest., 51, 2033-2039, 1972.

20. LANE, D.A., SCULLY, M.F., THOMAS, D.P., KAKKAR, V.V., WOOLF, I.W. and WILLIAMS, R.A. : Acquired dysfibrinogenemia in acute and chronic liver disease. Brit. J. Haemat., 35, 301-308, 1977.

21. LARGO, R., HELLER, V., STRAUB, W. : Detection of soluble intermediates of the fibrinogen-fibrin conversion using erythrocytes coated with fibrin monomers. Blood, 47, 991-1002, 1976.

22. LIPINSKI, B., GUREWICH, V., and LIPINSKA, I. : Thrombin time prolongation in cirrhosis in relation to enhanced fibrinogen degradation. Thromb. Research, 10, 185-187, 1977.

23. LIPINSKI, B., LIPINSKA, I., NOWAK, A., GUREWICH, V. : Abnormal fibrinogen heterogeneity and fibrinolytic activity in advanced liver disease. J. Lab. Clin. Med., 90, 187-194, 1977.

24. MANNUCCI, L., DIOGUARDI, N., DEL NINNO, E. & MANNUCCI, P.M., Value of thrombotest and antithrombin III in the assessment of liver function. Scandinavian Journal of Gastroenterology, 8, Suppl. 19, 103, 1973.

25. MARTINEZ, J., PALASCAK, J., PETERS, C. : Functional and metabolic properties of human asialofibrinogen. J. Lab. Clin. Med., 89, 367-377, 1977.

26. MARTINEZ, J., PALASCAK, J.E., KWASNIAK, D. : Abnormal sialic acid content of the dysfibrinogenaemia associated with liver disease. J. Clin. Invest. 61, 535-538, 1978.

27. MESTER, L. and SZABADOS, L. : Differences constitutionnelles entre les fragments glucidiques de fibrinogène humain normal et d'un fibrinogène anormal. Bull. Soc. Chim. Biol., 50, 2561-2575, 1978.

28. PALARETI, G., POGGI M., and COCCHERI, S. : Dual pattern in the dynamics of fibrinogen in liver cirrhosis : conversion to soluble fibrin and polymerisation defect. Vth International Congress on Thromboembolism. Bologna, Abstract p. 70, 1978.

29. PALASCAK, J.E. and MARTINEZ, J. : Dysfibrinogenemia associated with liver disease. J. Clin. Invest., 60, 89-92, 1977.

30. POLLER L. : Coagulation abnormalities in liver diseases. Recent Advance in blood coagulation. Edited by POLLER, Churchill Livingston, p 267-292, 1975.

31. RAKE, M.O., SHILKIN, K.B., WINCH, J., FLUTE, P.J., LEWIS, M.R. & WILLIAMS, R., Early and intensive therapy of intravascular coagulation in acute liver failure. Lancet, 2, 1215, 1971.

32. SAMAMA, M., SORIA, J., and SORIA, C. : Dysfibrinogénémies acquises. Discussion. Nouv. Rev. Fr. Hemat., 10, 666-669, 1970.

33. SAMAMA, M., SORIA, J., SORIA, C., Congenital and acquired dysdibrinogenemia. Recent advances in blood coagulation edited by POLLER. Churchill Livingstone, 313-336, 1975.

34. SCHWARTZ, M.L., PIZZO, S.V., HILL, R.L., and McKEE, P.A. : The effect of fibrin stabilisation factor on the sub-unit structure of human fibrin. J. Clin. Invest., 50, 1506-1509, 1971.

35. SERAFINI-CESSI, F. : Sialyltransferase activity in regererating rat liver. Biochem. J., 166, 381-386, 1977.

36. SHARON, N., LIS, H., Glycoproteins research booming on long-ignored ubiquitous compound. Chemical and Engineering news , 59, 21-44, 1981.

37. SORIA, J., COUPIER, J., SAMAMA, M.,TIXIER, P & BILSKI-PASQUIER, G. : Dysfibrinogenaemia without bleeding tendency with abnormal polymerization of fibrin monomers in a case of severe hepatitis. XII Congress of the International Society of Hematology, Abstract, p 180, 1968.

38. SORIA, J., SORIA, C., SAMAMA, M., COUPIER, J., GIRARD, M.L., BOUSSER, J., and BILSKI-PASQUIER, G. : Dysfibrinogénémies acquises dans les atteintes hépatiques sévères. Coagulation, 3, 37-44, 1970.

39. SORIA, J., SORIA, C., RYCKEWAERT, J.J., SAMAMA, M., THOMPSON, J.M., POLLER,L. : Study of acquired dysfibrinogenemia in liver disease. Thromb. Res., 19, 29-41, 1980.

40. SORIA, J.,SORIA, C., RODRIGUEZ, S.D, HORELOU, M., SAMAMA, M., BILSKI-PASQUIER, G. : Recherche de complexes solubles par un test d'hémagglutination. Application clinique. Presse Médicale, 6, 4045, 1977.

41. SORIA, J., SORIA, C., RYCKEWAERT, J.J. : A solid phase immunoenzymological assay for the measurement of human fibrinopeptide A. Thrombosis Research, 20, 425-435, 1980.

42. TYTGAT, GM, COLLEN, D & de VREKER, R.A. : la diathèse hémorragique en cas de cirrhose du foie. Coagulation, 1, 43, 1968.

43. TYTGAT, G.M., COLLEN, D & VERSTRAETE, M., Metabolism of fibrinogen in cirrhosis of the liver. Journal of Clinical Investigation, 50, 1690, 1971.

44. VERHAEGHE, R., VAN DAMME, B., MOLLA, A., and VERMYLEN, J. : Dysfibrinogenaemia associated with primary hepatoma. Scand. J. Haemat., 9, 451-458, 1972.

45. VERSTRAETE, M., VERMYLEN, J., COLLEN D. : Intravascular coagulation in liver disease. Ann. Rev. Med., 25, 447, 1974.

46. VON FELTEN, A., STRAUB, P.W., and FRICK, P.G. : Dysfibrinogenemia in a patient with primary hepatoma. First observation of an acquired abnormality of fibrin monomers. New Engl. J. Med., 208, (8), 405-409,1969.

47. WARREN, L., The thiobarbituric acid assay of sialic acid. J. Biol. Chem., 8,234-238, 1959.

48. WEINSTEIN, M.J., DEYKIN, D. : Quantitative abnormality of an α chain molecular weight form in the fibrinogen of cirrhotic patients. Br. J. Haemat. 40, 617-630,1978.

DISCUSSION LECTURE SORIA

Collen Do you think that carbohydrate abnormalities might also play a role in a prolonged thrombin time that you see in foetal fibrinogen?

Soria In foetal fibrinogen there is an increased level of sial acid.

Collen What about fibrinogen level adjustment in your assays?

Soria Usually fibrinogen level is not very low in our cases, so we have not to adjust the fibrinogen level, but in fibrin polymer regression curve we have to adjust fibrinogen level to compare with control to see if a clot is transfusant or not, but for thrombin-time we don't adjus

Soria You see, the thrombin clotting time is not so very prolonged as in a congenital disfibrinogenemia and we have noted no difference between a level of fibrinogen using immunological technique and using thrombin time.

Vinazzer Is the anticoagulant you have detected immunoglobulin?

Soria I don't know. We were not able to detect in what part of plasmaitis, because it is very difficult to isolate this anticoagulant. We were not able to isolate it; we have tried and we were unsuccessful.

PLATELET INVOLVEMENT IN THE HAEMOSTATIC FAILURE OF LIVER DISEASE

P. CAPEL

1. INTRODUCTION.

Besides local problems and coagulation deficiencies, which may lead to haemorrhage, both thrombocytopenia and platelet dysfunction may be involved in the haemostatic failure of patients suffering from liver disease.

2. THROMBOCYTOPENIA.

Thrombocytopenia is a common feature of liver disease. In liver cirrhosis, the frequency of this complication is high and varies from 37 to 77 % (3,5,9,II,I2,I8). Many causes have been evoked to explain this abnormality and will be briefly discussed.

Table 1. Causes of thrombocytopenia in liver failure.

- Splenomegaly.
- Disseminated intravascular coagulation.
- Bone marrow failure.
- Toxic effect of alcohol.
- Antiplatelet antibody and/or platelet associated IgG.

2.I. Splenomegaly

Excessive pooling of platelets by an enlarged spleen was described about 20 years ago by Aster (2). Labelled platelets, injected into patients, are distributed between two main pools : blood and spleen. In normal subjects, 50 to 80 % of transfused platelets are recovered in the blood. The remaining radioactivity is concentrated largely in the spleen. In splenomegalic patients, the recovery in the blood is lower, and more radioactivity is concentrated in the spleen.

The platelet splenic pool has been estimated by Penny and coworkers on surgically removed spleens (27). They have shown that the spleen content varied from 0.23 to 7.69 times the total circulating platelet mass. The total splenic platelet pool was higher than that, that can be calculated from the blood content of this organ.

2.2. Disseminated intravascular coagulation

Many patients with liver disease show abnormal coagulation tests suggestive of DIC. This problem has already been discussed by Dr. Collen and will not be reviewed here. The involvement of platelets in DIC during liver failure is suggested by their reduced half life observed by many authors (6, 12,15). However, in patients with stable liver cirrhosis, Scharf and collaborators were not able to show any elevation of βTG and PF4 levels, suggesting that no platelet activation occurs in those patients (33).

2.3. Bone marrow failure

Bone marrow failure can be observed in liver disease for various reasons.

- Folate deficiency is frequently encountered in liver disease, this resulting mainly from poor dietary intake and lowered storage capacity of the liver (37).

- Marrow aplasia is a rare but life-threatening complication of viral hepatitis (29).

- In animals, Siemensma and coworkers have shown that partial hepatectomy produces a lowering of circulating platelets (34). During experiments, platelet survival remained normal and no platelet pooling was observed. In vivo, labelling of platelets by radioactive selenomethionine was low, demonstrating a diminished production of platelets by the bone marrow.

These observations suggest that the liver may be involved in the regulation of platelet production. It has been suggested that the liver could be a source of thrombopoïetin.

In cirrhotic patients, Mayer and coworkers have observed a shortened maturation time of platelets, probably due to a disturbance in megakaryocyte maturation (22).

2.4. Effect of alcohol

Thrombocytopenia has been frequently observed during alcohol intake, even in the absence of abnormal liver function. Lindenbaum (I9) evaluated the frequency as I4 % in a group of non-cirrhotic alcoholics, regularly consulted. Cowan has observed a somewhat higher incidence in acutely ill alcoholics and a lower incidence in chronic alcoholics (9). In two studies with high controlled alcohol intake undertaken on a short number of patients, the frequency was approximately 50 % (7,20).

Bone marrow failure has been suggested by Sahud, who found that the platelet's size was diminished in alcoholics. Cowan has confirmed this hypothesis by showing that effective thrombopoïesis was diminished in such patients (7). It should be reminded that the vacuolated erythroblasts, seen in alcoholics, also suggest a toxic effect of ethanol on bone marrow. A lowering of circulating platelets during an ethanol infusion was observed in one patient. Labelled platelets injected prior to the experiment were also lowered. After 6 hours, the number of labelled and unlabelled platelets began to rise, suggesting a sequestration of platelets, although no organ could be implicated in this phenomenom (28).

2.5. Platelet antibodies

Antiplatelet antibodies and platelet associated IgG have been observed in some patients with acute and chronic hepatitis (I4,I7).

3. PLATELET DYSFUNCTION

Defective platelet function in liver disease was suspected a long time ago. Old studies using rather crude methods gave a somewhat higher incidence of these problems than more recent investigations. Following the latter methods, it seems that platelet dysfunction may be observed in approximately 50 % of th patients with chronic liver disease (3,5,I6, 21,31,35). The abnormality of platelet function in chronic liver disease has been shown, by Rubin and coworkers, to be proportional to the liver injury (3I). These authors have also shown a more severe failure of platelet function in acute liver disease (30,36). However, Langley has recently shown that platelet adhesiveness was increased in acute liver failure (I6).

Two main mechanisms have been proposed to explain this dysfunction of platelets.

3.1. Inhibition of platelet function by an extrinsic factor.

Thomas observed a correlation between delayed platelet aggregation and thrombin time in cirrhotic patients (35). The PPP of his patients showed an inhibitory effect on normal platelets aggregation. FDP seemed a good candidate to explain both abnormalities. The same inhibitory effect has been observed by Rubin, but the correlation between FDP level and delayed aggregation, although present, was not as good as that which Thomas found (31).

On the other hand, Ballard did not find any correlation between FDP and abnormal platelet aggregation in the same kind of patients (3). Owen, in patients with Wilson's disease, did not find any inhibitory effect of his patients platelet poor plasma on normal platelet aggregation (24).

3.2. Intrinsic platelet defect

Intrinsic platelet defect has been suggested in many studies (Table 2). As already mentionned, Sahud (32) has shown that platelets are smaller than normal in alcoholic patients. This observation has been confirmed by others in liver disease (31,36). As small platelets have been shown to function less well than large ones, this may partially explain the aggregation abnormalities observed.

Table 2. Intrinsic platelet abnormalities in liver disease

Weston et al (36) Rubin et al (31)	↓ platelet volume
Owen et al (25)	↑ cholesterol / phospholipid
	↓ arachidonic acid
Ahtee et al (1)	↓ serotonin uptake
Ordinas et al (23)	↓ glycoprotein I
Rubin et al (30)	vacuolisation microtubules

An elevation of platelet cholesterol has been observed by Owen (25). He also found a decrease in arachidonic acid. As the former abnormality is also found in type IIa hyper-lyoproteinemia, where platelet function is enhanced, this author attributed the defect of platelet function to the diminished arachidonic acid content.

Athee and collaborators found a reduced uptake of serotonin by washed platelets from cirrhotic patients (1).

It has been shown by Ordinas that glycoprotein I was lowered in liver cirrhosis (23).

Finally, Rubin and coworkers have shown abnormal ultrastructure of platelets in acute liver disease. These abnormalities consisted mainly in the presence of vacuoles and enhanced number of microtubules (30).

We have studied the electrophoretic mobility of factor VIII : RAg in liver cirrhosis. We have observed, like others, an abnormal anodal electrophoretic mobility of factor VIII : RAg in plasma but not in platelets, suggesting a plasmatic degradation of this factor (Fig. 1).

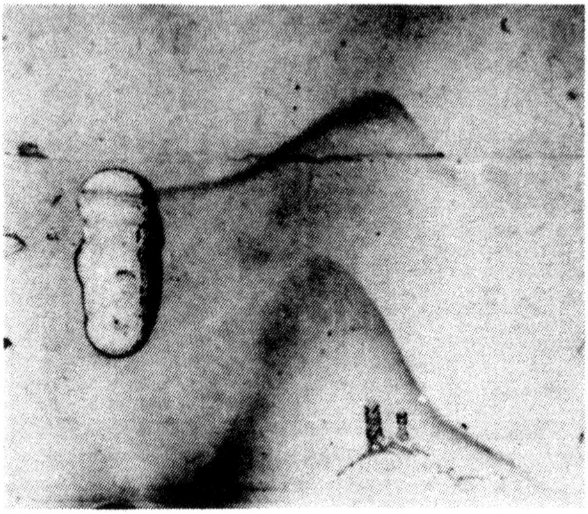

FIGURE 1 : Crossed immunoelectrophoresis of factor VIII R : Ag in the plasma (upper precipitation line) and in the platelets (lower precipitation line) of a cirrhotic patient.

On the other hand, we observed a high concentration of factor VIII : RCF in those patients, which rules out any implication of this factor in their bleeding problems.

It thus seems that,in spite of the fact that FDP may play some inhibitory role, the main defect of platelet function is due to an intrinsic abnormality. The question which then arisis is how this abnormality occurs (Table 3). It has already been mentionned that bone marrow produces less platelets in liver disease. Qualitative disturbances have also been observed the shortened maturation time of megakaryocytes suggested by Mayer in cirrhotic patients has already been mentioned (22). In the study of Siemensma, a decrease in size and ploïdy of the megakaryocytes have been observed in rats after partial hepatectomy (34).

Table 3. Possible causes of platelets abnormalities in liver disease

- Abnormal thrombopoiesis	
. Siemensma et al (34) :	↓ size and ploïdy of megakaryocytes after partial hepatectomy.
. Mayer et al (22) :	↓ maturation time of platelets.
- DIC	
. Pareti et al (26) :	storage pool disease
- Splenomegaly	
. Freedman and Karpathin (10) :	preferential sequestration of large platelets by the spleen.
- Alcohol	
. Haut and Cowan :	↓ platelet function in vivo and in vitro

Acquired storage pool disease has been observed in DIC by Pareti (26). A possible cause of these abnormalities is an activation of platelets to release their content by agents like thrombin and plasmin.

In animal studies, Freedman and coworkers have observed that the spleen preferentially sequestrated large platelets, leaving thus smaller and less active platelets in the circulating blood (10).

Alcohol not only induces thrombopenia but also inhibits platelet aggregation in vivo and in vitro as it has been shown by Haut and Cowan. These authors have observed numerous biochemical abnormalities of platelets induced by ethanol : diminished production of CO_2 after stimulation by adrenalin, decreased in glucose utilisation after thrombin stimulation, decreased production of cAMP.

4. CONCLUSIONS

The frequence of thrombocytopenia and platelet disfunction is high in liver disease. The causes of both abnormalities are poorly understood and are multiple and variable from one patient to an other. Except for severe thrombopenia, the clinical importance of those disorders is difficult to assess. but it seems that platelet dysfunction plays a more important role in acute liver disease.

A better knowledge of the mechanisms involved will lead to a better therapeutical approach to those problems and give more information on the role played by the liver in thrombopoïesis and platelet function.

REFERENCES

1. Athee L, Briley M, Raisman R, Lebrec D and Langer S. Reduced uptake of serotonin but unchanged ^{3}H-imipramine binding in the platelets from cirrhotic patients. Life Sci. 29 : 2323-2329, I98I
2. Aster R. Pooling of Platelets in the Spleen : Role in the Pathogenesis of "Hypersplenic" Thrombocytopenia. J. Clin. Invest. 45 : 645-657, I966
3. Ballard H, Aaron J. Platelet Aggregation in Portal Cirrhosis Arch. Int. Med. I36 : 3I6-3I9, I976
4. Breddin K. Hämorrhagische Diathesen bei Lebererkrankungen unter besonderer Berücksichtigung der Thrombocytenfunktion Acta haemat. 27 : 1-16, I962
5. Cortet P, Klepping C, Devant J, Lebel J.P., Jacquot B. Le facteur3plaquettaire au cours des cirrhoses alcooliques. Etude de l'adhésivité in vivo par le test de Borchgrevink. Arch. Mal. App. Digestif. 53 : I04I-I045, I964
6. Cooney D, Smith A. The Pathophysiology of Hypersplenic Thrombocytopenia. Arch. Intern. Med. I2I : 332-337, I968
7. Cowan D. Thrombokinetic studies in alcohol-related thrombocytopenia. J. Lab. Clin. Med. 8I : 64-76, I973
8. Cowan D. Effect of alcoholism on Haemostasis. Semin. Hematol. I7 : I37-I47, I980
9. Donaldson G, Davies S, Darg A, Richmond J. Coagulation factors in chronic liver disease. J. Clin. Pathol. 22 : I99-204, I969
IO. Freedman M, Karpatkin S. Heterogeneity of Rabbit Platelets. V. Preferential splenic sequestration of megathrombocytes Brit. J. Haematol. 3I : 255-262, I975
II. Frick P. Thrombocytopenie und Lebercirrhose. Schweiz. Med. Wschr. 37 : 407-4I3, I967
I2. Gehrmann G, Elbers C. Thrombopenisches Hyperspleniesyndrom bei splenomegaler Leberzirrhose. Deutsche Medizinische Wochenschrift 27 : I429-I432, I970
I3. Haut M, Cowan D. The Effect of Ethanol on Hemostatic properties of Human Blood Platelets. Am. J. Med. 56 : 22-23, I974

I4. Karpatkin S, Strick N, Karpatkin M, Siskind G. Cumulative Experience in the Detection of Antiplatelet Antibody in 234 Patients with Idiopathic Thrombocytopenic Purpura, Systemic Lupus Erythematosus and Other Clinical Disorders. Am. J. Med. 52 : 776-785, I972
I5. Kummer H, Egger G. Pathogenese des Thrombopenie bei Leberzirrhose. Schweiz. Med. Wschr. IOI : I8I6-I8I7, I97I
I6. Langley P, Hughes R, Williams R. Platelet Adhesiveness to Glass Beads in Liver Disease. Acta haemat. 67 : I24-I27, I982
I7. Leone G, Agostini A, Mango G, Landolfi R, Valori V, Bizzi B. Megathrombocytes, Platelet Regeneration Time and Platelet-Associated IgG in Idiopathic Thrombocytopenic Purpura and in Thrombocytopenia Associated with Chronic Liver Disease. Acta haemat. 65 : 40-47, I98I
I8. Levrat M, Truchot R. Le rôle de la thrombopénie dans les hémorragies des cirrhoses du foie. Arch. Mal. Appar. Dig. 5I : I394-I404, I962
I9. Lindenbaum J, Hargrove R. Thrombocytopenia in Alcoholics. Ann. Intern. Med. 68 : 526-532,I968
20. Lindenbaum J, Lieber C. Hematologic Effects of Alcohol in man in the Absence of Nutritional Deficiency. New Engl. J. Med. 28I : 333-338, I969
2I. Mandel E, Lazerson J. Thrombasthenia in Liver Disease. New Engl. J. Med. 265 : 56-6I, I96I
22. Mayer M, Herrmann I, Kempgens U, Queisser W. In vivo Labeling of Platelets with 75 Se-Selenomethionine in Patients with Hepatic Cirrhosis and Thrombocytopenia. Thrombos. Haemostas. (Stuttg.) 37 : 47-52,I977
23. Ordinas A, Marogall S, Castillo R, Nurden A. A glycoprotein I defect in the platelets of three patients with severe cirrhosis of the liver. Thromb. Res. I3 : 297-302, I978
24. Owen C, Goldstein N, Bowie E. Platelet Function and Coagulation in Patients with Wilson Disease. Arch. Intern. Med. I36 : I48-I52, I976
25. Owen J, Hutton R, Day R, Bruckdorger K, Mc Intyre N. Platelet lipid composition and platelet aggregation in human liver disease. J. Lip. Res. 22 : 423-430, I98I
26. Pareti F, Capitano A, Mannucci P. Acquired Storage Pool Disease in Platelets During Disseminated Intravascular Coagulation. Blood 48 : 5II-5I5, I976
27. Penny R, Rozenberg M, Firkin B. The Splenic Platelet Pool. Blood 27 : I-I6, I966
28. Post R, Desforges J. Thrombocytopenic Effect of Ethanol Infusion. Blood 3I : 344-347, I968
29. Rosner F. Aplastic anaemia and viral hepatitis. Lancet ii,I080, I970
30. Rubin M, Weston M, Bullock G, Roberts J, Langley P, White S, Williams R. Abnormal Platelet Function and Ultrastructure in Fulminant Hepatic Failure. Quart. J. Med. I83 : 339-352, I977

3I. Rubin M, Weston M, Langley P, White Y, Williams R. Platelet Function in Chronic Liver Disease. Dig. Dis. Sci. 24 : I97-202, I979
32. Sahud M. Platelet Size and Number in Alcoholic Thrombocytopenia. New. Engl. J. Med. 286 : 355-356, I972
33. Scharf R, Schramm W, Heisig S, Schneider W. Does chronic Disseminated intravascular coagulation (DIC) cause Thrombocytopenia in patients with stable liver cirrhosis ? Haemostasis I2 : 39,I982 (Abstract)
34. Siemensma N, Bathal P, Penington D. The effect of massive liver resection on platelet kinetics in the rat. J. Lab. Clin. Med. : 86 : 8I7-833, I975
35. Thomas D. Abnormalities of platelet aggregation in patients with alcoholic cirrhosis. Ann. N.Y. Acad. Sci. 20I : 243-250, I972
36. Weston P, Langley P, Rubin M, Hanid A, Mellon P, Williams R. Platelet function in fulminant hepatic failure and effect of charcoal haemoperfusion. Gut I8 : 897-902, I977
37. Wintrobe M. Clinical Hematology. Lea and Febiger, Philadelphia, Eight Edition, 58I, I98I.

DISCUSSION LECTURE CAPEL

Soria I would like to tell you a story, I am glad to tell you that abnormal fibrinogen will not induce an abnormal platelet aggregation, because we've tried plateled co-factor activity in platelet aggregation of our abnormal fibrinogen, and it is normal or little increased.

Mannucci How often do you find in patients with severe liver disease a prolonged bleeding time?

Capel In chronic liver disease, the bleeding-time is quite often normal, but in acute liver disease Rubin studied six patients and the most of them had a prolonged bleeding-time.

Samama I would like to make a comment. Of course, in his excellent review Mannucci has pointed out also this dicrepancy, but I think in your review, you were talking about the DUKE-method, which is not very sensitive. If you use a sensitive method, I think there would be more often an increase in the bleeding-time in this kind of patients, especially when the platelet count is lower than 100,000. So we have also to take into account the methodology. But of course the Duke bleeding time is usually normal. Do you agree?

Mannucci Yes, I think that we would agree with him that in chronic liver disease bleeding time is not very often off the proportion of the number of platelets you're taking into account, according to the Hawker formula. I don't want to put a lot of emphasis to the abnormalities of aggregation. I'm not sure that it is a platelet dysfunction.

Vinazzer There may be some practical problems with platelet aggregation in patients with severe liver disease. In order to compare aggregation, first you have to standardize, and you have also to standardize the platelet count around at 200,000. Now, when you have a platelet count between 50,000 and 70,000 in a patient with cirrhosis, you have a very hard time to get a patient which has a platelet count of 200,000.

Verstraete Normal individuals, without liver disease, can have an induced thrombocytopenia due to alcolhol. Do you know i patients with liver disease have an increased sensitivi to alcohol in terms of induced thombocytopenia?

Capel I don't know.

THE SIGNIFICANCE OF SEVERAL COAGULATION TESTS IN THE EVALUATION OF THE RISK OF BLEEDING

M. SAMAMA

Coagulation tests are widely used in liver diseases in the evaluation of hepatic insufficiency. They are obligatory in the assessment of the risk of bleeding in patients submitted to surgical procedures such as liver biopsy, minor or major surgery.

In the assessment of hemorrhagic tendency of patients with chronic liver disease, it is important to discriminate bleeding from the gastro-intestinal tract associated with oesophagial varices and/or superficial erosions. For most authors coagulation defects play a minor role in the mechanism of these bleeding episodes.

On the contrary, ecchymotic purpura, epistaxis, bleeding and ecchymosis at ponction sites and post traumatic bleeding are mainly due to different alterations of haemostasis. These alterations are complex and multifaceted as stated recently by Bick (2) and by many authors (3,4,6,9,IO,II,I2,I3,I4,I5,I6).

- Decreased and/or defective synthesis of coagulation proteins including coagulation inhibitors such as Antithrombin III (AT III) and Protein C.
- Quantitative platelet and/or qualitative platelet defects.
- Vascular dysfunction due to increased capillary permability, vitamin deficiency and excess of circulating oestrogens.
- Primary or secondary hyperfibrinogenolysis.
- Intravascular coagulation possibly after some triggering events.

The pathogenesis of these possible haemostatic abnormalities has been identified through numerous studies dealing with this subject.

Five main different mechanisms have been suggested :

- Failure of synthesis of most coagulation proteins and of
  - important factors in the fibrinolytic system;
  - Production of abnormal factors such as abnormal fibrinogen and the PIVKAs;
  - Impaired clearance of tissue plasminogen activator and of actived coagulation proteins;
  - Increased catabolism such as in disseminated intravascular coagulation (DIC);
  - Extravascular losses of coagulation proteins.

Concerning the failure of synthesis, it is interesting to note that the decrease in the plasma level of natural inhibitors such as AT III and Protein C might compensate the decrease in coagulation factors such as prothrombin and Factor V.

This equilibrium could explain why severe bleeding and thrombosis may not occur despite important alterations of haemostasis.

Increased fibrinolytic activity is frequently observed in patients with liver cirrhosis. It has been attributed to an increase in plasma tissue plasminogen activator due to an impaired clearance of this activator by the liver. A reduction in alpha-$_2$-antiplasmin and in Histidin Rich Glycoprotein may also play a role. However, reduction in plasminogen concentration can counter balance blood hyperfibrinolytic activity (I, I7, I9).

Finally the problem of DIC in liver disease has been discussed in the same journal by Collen.

More than one mechanism is probably frequently involved in the resulting plasma levels of coagulation proteins as illustrated by two examples : firstly, fibrinogen and secondly, Factor V. A decreased synthesis of fibrinogen is observed in severe liver disease. In patients with cirrhosis of the liver and DIC an increased catabolism of fibrinogen has been demonstrated. Furthermore, an increased fibrinogen turnover and/or the production of an abnormal fibrinogen (acquired dysfibrinogenemia) have been found in patients with liver cirrhosis. The role of acquired dysfibrinogenemia in the bleeding syndrome has not been unequivocally shown (8, 18,20).

A decrease in Factor V plasma level in patients with liver disease may have different origins : decreased synthesis and increased catabolism due to DIC. Moreover Factor V is often decreased in patients with splenomegaly. The mechanism of this alteration is obscur.

The mechanism of thrombocytopenia in liver cirrhosis is not well understood. Three different mechanisms have been advocated :

- Increased splenic sequestration in connection with splenomegaly, present in many patients;
- Increased consumption due to classical DIC or more probably to a more complex mechanism involving the role of abnormal endovascular surfaces and local stasis in the liver (13);
- Decreased production is another possible mechanism, since alcoholism and folate deficiency can decrease platelet production,

However in a recent work, Stein and Harker in a very well conducted study, were able to demonstrate a reduction in mean platelet survival and an increase in splenic sequestration of platelets in patients with chronic liver disease (5). Finally, combination of different intricated mechanisms might occur frequently, resulting sometimes in a normal platelet count altough platelet production is abnormal (21).

Finally, different tests are routinely used for the screening of these haemostatic changes in liver diseases. The main tests which we recommend are listed below :

- Platelet count and bleeding time;
- Prothrombin and partial thromboplastin time;

- Fibrinogen plasma level and thrombin clotting time;
- FDP and fibrinolytic activity evaluation.

As pointed out by Mannucci, these broad-spectrum tests such as PT and PTT are generally more useful than the specific assays of individual clotting factors, for the evaluation of hepatic insufficiency and for the assessment of the risk of bleeding.(I3)

Let us consider briefly the evaluation of hepatic insufficiency.

In a previous work in I975 (4), we studied 60 patients with liver cirrhosis. We used 3 differents criteria of hepatic insufficiency :

- Albumin $<$ 35 g/l;
- Cholesterol $<$ I.5 g/l;
- An abnormal BSP clearance, being the third criteria.

9 patients had no criteria, 23 one, 20 two and finally 7 patients had 3 criterias.

Table 1. Relationship between coagulation tests and liver insufficiency.

	n	PT (%)	VII+X (%)	V (%)	Fgen (g/L)	Plat	ATIII (sec)	TCT (P/C)
0 criteria	9	64	7I	68	4.4	229	79	I.I3
1 criteria	23	46	40	48	2.4	I05	48	I.35
2 criteria	20	47	43	49	2.4	II4	42	I.33
3 criteria	7	37	30	43	2.0	80	35	I.46

This table shows the results obtained for seven different coagulation tests. Statistically significant differences were found between the results of patients with I and with 0 and 3 criterias. No statistical difference was found between the patients with I and 2 criterias and in the groups of patients with 2 or 3 criterias.

In the same study, we analysed the relationship between coagulation tests and hemorrhagic syndrome. We have selected 42 patients with well documented liver cirrhosis and without gastro-intestinal bleeding. Among these 42 patients, IO had an hemorrhagic syndrome while 32 had no bleeding episodes.

Table 2. Coagulation tests and hemorrhagic syndrome in liver cirrhosis.

Hemor-rhage	n	V (%)	VII+X (%)	II (%)	PTT (P/C)	I (g/l)	Plgen (g/l)	Plat	r+k (mm)	am (mm)
+	IO	43	29	37	49	I.9	28	56	42	37
-	32	53	5I	53	44	3.0	54	I48	30	32
p		*	***	**	**	***	***	****	****	****

* $p < 0.05$ ** $p < 0.02$ *** $p < 0.0I$ **** $p < 0.00I$

Hemor-rhage	n	PT (%)	TCT (P/C)	FDP (µg/l)	ATIII (sec)	Eugl. Clt I20 min	+ Eth. g.t.
+	IO	4I	I.45	67	38	4	I
-	32	5I	I.32	47	60	I6	I
p		ns	ns	ns	ns	ns	ns

ns : not significant

Among I5 different parameters, 9 were able to discriminate between these two groups of patients. 6 parameters gave no statistically significant results. It is interesting to note that thromboelastographic results were very discriminant although the usefulness of this test is not generally accepted.

However, we must admit that we could not find any single test which could predict the risk of bleeding even if we try to make a score including different tests. In a more recent study, including alpha-$_2$-antiplasmin and Histidin Rich Glycoprotein (H.R.G.P.) determinations, no close relationship was evidenced between the coagulation tests and the bleeding risk. Platelet count was probably the less dissapointing test as regards the assessment of hemorrhagic tendency in both studies.

However, dispite the results of this study, clinical experience suggests that if the following haemostatic changes are not present, the risk of bleeding is minimal. These limits are : (7)

- Platelet count over 80,000/mm^3;
- Without prolonged bleeding time. It is interesting to note that bleeding time in patients with liver cirrhosis is often shorter than expected from the results of platelet count (I3);
- Prothrombin time activity>40 %;
- Fibrinogen>I.5 g/l;
- No increase of FDP, no decrease below 90 minutes of ELT. These last parameters are important if we consider that low grade DIC can become fulminant after some triggering event such as a general anesthaesia and surgery in patients with liver cirrhosis.

In some patients with heamostatic alterations submitted to surgical procedures, management of hemostatic failure must take into account the complex mechanism of the haemostatic defect in patients with chronic liver disease. Substitutive therapy is based, for every coagulation factor, on their half-life; and on the level required for hemostasis.

Table 3. From BLOOM (I98I) (3)

	Half -Life	Level Required For Haemostasis	Recovery
Prothrombin (II)	50 h	40 %	-
Proconvertin (VII)	3 to 6 h	IO %	Almost complete
Stuart Factor (X)	24 to 72 h	20 - 30 %	-
Proaccelerin (V)	I5 to 24 h	20 %	50 %
Fibrinogen (I)	4 days	I g/l	-

Fresh frozen plasma is said to be the most suitable agent for this group of patients, but very large volumes of plasma are required in order to obtain a satisfactory correction of the clotting tests.

Prothrombin complex concentrates are more effective but their use is limited by the risk of triggering DIC and by the risk of hepatitis. Concomitant administration of heparin or of AT III concentrates may reduce the potential risk of DIC.

Short therapy is recommended and is specially useful just before liver biopsy or minor surgical procedure. The use of E. A.C.A. or Tranexamic acid as an antifibrinolytic drug, is not recommended unless active hyperfibrinolysis is demonstrated. A short term treatment must be prefered to long term therapy since antifibrinolytic drugs are contraindicated in DIC and can predispose to thrombosis.

Platelet concentrates are very useful in patients with severe thrombocytopenia undergoing surgery, although the increase in platelet count is moderate, since platelets are rapidly removed from the circulation.

Vitamin K of course, is administrated if vitamin deficiency due to malabsorption is present.

The problem of heparin and AT III concentrates in patients with DIC is discussed by Collen and is also dealt with by Ten Cate in the same journal.

Finally, in conclusion, I would like to give two examples in order to illustrate these therapeutical problems.

Mr. MOI... is a 46 year old man with post-hepatitic liver cirrhosis. He must undergo a cholecystectomy. His hemostatic profile shows a normal bleeding time with the Duke's method and a very prolonged bleeding time with Simplate's method. PT and PTT are abnormal, as well as his thrombin clotting time. Euglobulin lysis time is very short.

Table 4. Mr. MOI... 46 y.o. Liver cirrhosis (post-hepatitis) ⟶ Cholecystectomy.

Bleeding time : Duke 5 min., Simplate > I5 min.

Platelet count : 43,000/μl

PT : 53 % - V : 35 % - VII + X : 50 % - II : 40 %

PTT : 50 sec. / Control 36 sec.

TCT : 25 sec. / Control 20 sec.

Fibrinogen : 2.I0 g/l

Euglobulin C.L.T. : 40 min. (Nl I80 min.)

F.D.P. : 2 μg/ml

TEG : r = 2I mm - K = I2 mm - am = 35 mm

During surgery, 5 million units of Kunitz inhibitor, fresh frozen plasma and platelet concentrates were perfused; the plasma and platelet concentrates were continued 24 hrs after surgery. No important modification of the coagulation tests was obtained and no abnormal bleeding encountered.

Table 5.	D_O	D_O Evening	D_1	D_2
Platelet count (/mm^3)	43,000	56,000	50,000	30,000
Prothromb. activity (%)	53	55	46	48
Factors V (%)	35	48	--	40
VII + X (%)	52	50	--	30
II (%)	40	50	--	50
PTT (sec.)	43/C.37	44/C.40	5I/C.38	45/C.38
Fibrinogen (g/ml)	2.I0	2.I0	2.40	2.50
F.D.F. (μg/ml)	2	-	8	I6
Euglobulin CLT (h.)	40 min.	2 h 45	2	2 h 40

In the second example, a 67 y.o. woman with severe liver cirrhosis, undergoes hip surgery. A fall down in platelet count and in some coagulation proteins is associated with normal fibrinolytic activity.

Fresh frozen plasma (3 units) and platelet concentrates

(IO units) were administered per and post-operatively and no bleeding was encountered.

Table 6. Mrs. CHA... 67 y.o. Liver cirrhosis - Hip surgery

	D_0	D_1	D_2	D_5
Platelet count (/mm^3)	60,000	88,000	68,000	--
Prothrom.activity (%)	46	47	44	39
Factors V (%)	40	52	--	36
VII + X (%)	36	35	--	30
II (%)	55	70	--	50
PTT (sec.)	44/C.35	--	--	52/C/40
Fibrinogen (g/l)	3.IO	2.40	2.I5	2.IO
F.D.P. (µg/ml)	I6	I6	--	8
Euglobulin CLT (h.)	> 20	3 h 30	--	7

In conclusion, haemostatic changes are frequently observed in liver cirrhosis. They are associated or not with bleeding. In the absence of bleeding, it does not seem necessary to correct these changes since an equilibrium may be present at a level different from normal state : low coagulation factor levels, associated with low inhibitor levels. However, if a surgical procedure or a liver biopsy is required, a treatment should be undertaken. (7, I3).

The relationship between haemostatic changes and risk of bleeding is not clear but one can define values which may constitute limits above which the risk is minimal.

The management of haemostatic failure is well documented. Platelet concentrates and fresh frozen plasma are often effective in preventing bleeding in patients submitted to surgical procedures such as liver biopsy, minor or major surgery.

REFERENCES

1. Aoki N, Yamanak T. 1978. α_2-plasmin inhibitor levels in liver diseases. Clin. Chim. Acta, 84, 99-105.

2. Bick RL. 1983. Disseminated intravascular coagulation and related syndromes. In : Alterations of hemostasis in chronic liver diseases. RCR Press Inc. Baca Raton, Florida, 121-125.

3. Brozovic M. 1982. Pathogenesis of haemostatic abnormalities in liver diseases. In : Haemostasis and Thrombosis, Blom A, Thomas D. Eds. Churchill Livinstone, 422-428.

4. Conard J, Certin M, Samama M, Opolon P. 1975. Les troubles de la coagulation au cours des cirrhoses, et leur traitement. J. Franç. Gastro-Ent. Masson Ed., Paris, 188-203.

5. Couinaud C. 1979. Action de la splénectomie sur les troubles plaquettaires des cirrhotiques. Chirur. 105, 380-383.

6. Couinaud C. 1980. Introduction à l'étude de l'hémostase chez le cirrhotique. Sem. Hôp. Paris 29(32), 1323-1329.

7. Forestier F, Boisson J., Samama M. 1975. Contre-indications de la ponction biopsie hépatique. Sem. Hôp. Paris 51(46), 2815-2817.

8. Francis JL, Armstrong DJ. 1982. Acquired dysfibrinogenemia in liver disease J. Clin. Pathol. 35, 667-672.

9. Guillin MC, Menache D, Barge D, Rueff B, Fauvert R, Curé R, Dosse J, Lorin J. 1971. Les troubles de l'hémostase au cours des hépatites virales graves. Etude clinique, anatomique et biologique. Ann. Med. Intern. 122(5), 605-612.

10. Larrieu MJ. 1976. Les troubles de l'hémostase et de la coagulation chez les cirrhotiques. Revue Prat. 26(51), 3651-3657.

11. Lechner K, Niesser H, Thaler E. 1977. Coagulation abnormalities in liver disease. Semin. Thromb. Haemostas. 4, 422-428.

12. Lurie B, Creter D. 1981. Coagulation studies for severe liver disease detection in a gastro-enterologic department. Digestion 21, 244-247.

13. Mannucci P, Mari D. 1981. Haemostasis and liver disease. Hematologica 66(2), 233-248.

14. Marchal G, Samama M, Prost RJ. 1960. Etude de la coagulation et de l'hémostase dans 74 cas de cirrhoses. Sang 8 XXXI, 704-715.

15. Nilsson IM. 1964. Coagulation studies in liver disease. Thrombos. Diathes. Haemorrh. 11, 51-58.

16. Rajni MU, Lewis JH, Spero JA, Hasiba U. 1982. Bleeding and coagulation abnormalities in alcohol cirrhosis liver disease. Alcoholism : Clinical Experimental Research 6(2), 267-274.

17. Saito H, Goodnough LT, Boyle JM, Heimburger N. 1981. Reduced Histidin Rich Glycoprotein levels in plasma of patients with advanced liver cirrhosis. Amer. J. Med. 73, 179-182.

18. Samama M, Soria C, Soria J. 1970. Dysfibrinogénémies acquises. Nouv. Revue Franç. Hématol. 10(5), 666-669.

19. Samama M, Schlegel N., Cazenave B, Horellou MH, Conard J, Castel M, Douenias R. α_2-antiplasmin assay : amidolytic and immunological method. Critical evaluation. Results in a clinical material. In : Synthetic Substrates in Clinical Blood Coagulation Assays. Lijnen HR, Collen D, Verstraete M. Eds., 93-98.

20. Soria J, Soria C, Ryckewaert JJ, Samama M, Thomson JM, Poller L. 1980. Study of acquired dysfibrinogenemia in liver disease. Thrombos Res. 19, 29-41.

21. Stein SF, Harker LA. 1982. Kinetic and functional studies of platelets fibrinogen and plasminogen in patients with hepatic cirrhosis. J. Lab. Clin. Med. 99, 217-230.

DISCUSSION LECTURE SAMAMA

Mannucci I would like to say that I agree with most of your comments. I would like to make two comments on the screening test and the other one to replacement therapy with prothrombin complex concentrates. The most frequent problem in term of surgery in connection with bleeding is that patients with liver disease need a liver biopsy. The operations of course can happen but they are not very frequent at least in our hands. The le-Veen shunt is done less and less. So, the main problem is liver biopsy procedure. We gave low importance to the bleeding time rather than to the clotting tests and more than to the clinic counts, because we have found that patients with 40,000 platelets, may have a normal bleeding time. In this case, we do liver biopsy in respect of the number of platelet counts. The test must be more sensitive than Duke bleeding time, the simplate method. The problem will be the correction of the coagulation abnormalities with prothrombin complex concentrates. You say that the main risk is the thromboembolism. I really don't think that this is the main risk particularly providing that you give also some plasma, plasma-inhibitors or maybe antithombin III itself together with concentrates. The major risk with these concentrates is that of giving to this patients viral hepatitis, which is really delicate for some patients with liver failure. So, until the concentrates are hepatitis safer, or hepatitis free, than which are now prepared, there is no reason to use these concentrates for liver biopsy.

Samama I agree but I think that we must agree that if you perform a Duke bleeding-time you'll have almost normally many patients with low platelet counts as you said 30,000. But I am quite sure that in these patients, if you perform a 'simplate', it will be prolonged like in the patient I have shown.

Mannucci I said the Duke bleeding-time should not be done and a more sensitive test should be done.

Soria I would like to make a comment about liver biopsy. When the hemostatic function is very bad in liver cirrhosis, we have perhaps to perform a liver biopsy by trans-jugular, so the risk of bleeding is less intense.

David Is the euglobulin lysis time frequently abnormal in your patients?

Samama In our cases, the euglobulin lysis time was very short. In very previous studies, we have found some patients with liver cirrhosis during major surgery with a very increased fibinolytic activity.

CLINICAL MANIFESTATIONS OF THE HAEMOSTATIC FAILURE IN ACUTE AND CHRONIC LIVER DISEASE

ROGER WILLIAMS
and I.R.CROSSLEY

Severe bleeding in acute or chronic liver disease may result from lesions localised to the gastrointestinal tract, most commonly oesophageal or gastric varices and erosions. Haemorrhage from frank peptic ulceration can also occur but is much less frequent. In the terminal stages of liver failure generalised bleeding into the skin and mucous membranes is seen. Petroperitoneal haemorrhage, bleeding from the nasopharynx, bronchial free, uterus and bladder occur occasionally whilst cerebral haemorrhage is rare. Less common, but important, septicaemia may contribute to haemostatic failure. Procedures such as ascites reinfusion or insertion of a peritoneovenous shunt are well recognised as exacerbating the haemostatic defect. It is important to recognise that spontaneous bleeding into the peritoneal cavity may come from a liver tumour. Surgery is particularly hazardous for the cirrhotic in the presence of an abnormal coagulation profile; and procedures such as liver biopsy can be followed by bleeding even when the haemostatic profile is normal.

Fulminant Hepatic Failure

The incidence of clinically significant haemorrhage in early series of patients with fulminant hepatic failure varies from 41% to 73% (1-3). Death is not infrequently due to haemorrhage. In one representative series from the Liver Unit, King's College Hospital (4) in 1975, major bleeding was the principal cause of death in 28 (29%) of 96 patients with fulminant hepatic failure and in 89%

of cases originated from the gastrointestinal tract (Table 1). In a further study from the same Unit, the source of upper gastrointestinal bleeding at gastrointestinal endoscopy was found to be oesophageal and/or gastric erosions in 94% of cases. The cause of these mucosal lesions is uncertain, however gastric acid appears to be required for their development.

An initial study of 25 patients with fulminant hepatic failure showed that prophylactic 4-hourly administration of antacids did not affect the frequency of bleeding from erosions (5) but was probably related to failure to maintain a high intragastric pH (Fig. 1). Larger doses of antacid which maintain intragastric pH above 5 have shown a reduction in the frequency of haemorrhage, however such therapy could be dangerous in these patients who frequently develop renal failure and metabolic alkalosis. Following the introduction of H_2 receptor antagonists, continuous suppression of gastric acid secretion resulted in almost complete elimination of gastrointestinal bleeding - one of 26 treated patients bled compared to 13 (54%) of 24 controls (Fig. 1). The survival of patients who did not bleed was strikingly different from those who did. Gastrointestinal haemorrhage is now uncommon since the prophylactic use of cimetidine. Although fulminant hepatic failure is associated with a profound disturbance of coagulation, there is not a close correlation between the latter and the frequency of gastro intestinal bleeding. Nevertheless a challenge to haemostasis presented by a defect in vascular integrity is more likely to result in bleeding in patients in whom haemostasis is compromised.

Studies have evaluated the value of coagulation factor replacement either as fresh frozen plasma or factor concentrates in the prevention of the bleeding diathesis (5,6). Large volumes of fresh frozen plasma are required and the prothrombin time is difficult to correct

Figure I. Results of a controlled trial in which antacids or cimetidine was given prophylactically in patients with fulminant hepatic failure showing marked decrease in subsequent bleeding with the latter drug (from Macdougall et al).

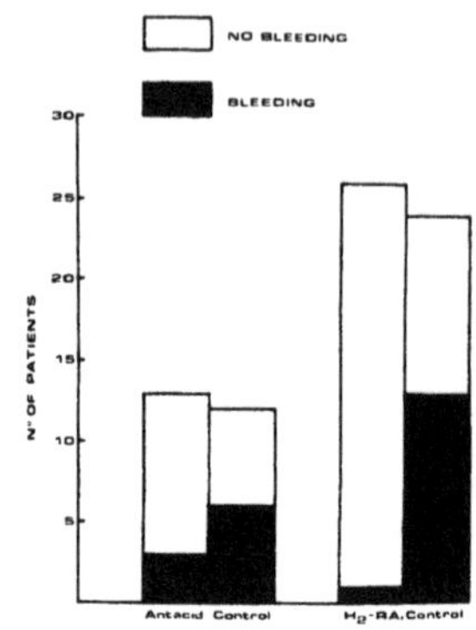

Figure 2. Results of controlled trial in fulminant hepatic failure in which fresh frozen plasma was given to correct coagulation deficit. No decrease in subsequent bleeding observed.

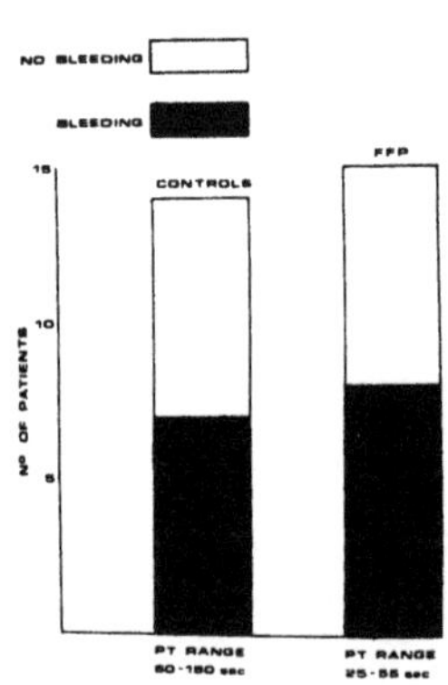

completely. The biological survival of coagulation factors is short and frequent administration is necessary. Circulatory overload or electrolyte imbalance may be easily precipitated and 300 ml 6-hourly is close to the limits of tolerance during continuous administration. A controlled trial involving 29 patients in which fresh frozen plasma was given prophylactically and a three-fold reduction in prothrombin time achieved showed no decrease in the frequency of subsequent bleeding (Fig. 2). Nevertheless, fresh frozen plasma remains a mainstay of treatment in any actively bleeding patient.

Concentrates of the Vitamin K dependant factors are highly potent and circumvent the haemodynamic problems associated with fresh frozen plasma. They may transmit viral hepatitis and also contain activated coagulation factors which could exacerbate intravascular coagulation. In one controlled trial of clotting factor concentrates in fulminant hepatic failure, three of five patients so treated developed major bleeding and died, two developed clinical evidence of disseminated intravascular coagulation (DIC). Laboratory evidence of DIC progressed in all patients in both patient groups but was less marked in those receiving heparin as well as the factor concentrate (6).

Early studies in which thrombocytopaenia, hypofibrinogenaemia, fibrin degradation products and increased plasma disappearance of ^{125}I fibrinogen suggested that DIC was a common event and heparin could have a place in therapy. The only controlled trial in the literature (7) showed no benefit and the true incidence of disseminated intravascular coagulation remains controversial.

Thrombocytopaenia and qualitative changes in platelet function are common in fulminant hepatic failure. Circulating platelets are already activated in these patients as judged by increased plasma levels of B-thromboglobulin, and a poor response to aggregating agents. Despite these changes, serial charcoal haemoperfusion even with polymer coating of the charcoal is associated with platelet clumping and unacceptable platelet losses. Increased platelet adhesiveness occurs in these patients and may predispose to such changes. The cause is unknown but may in part be related to elevated levels of Factor VIII. Heparin, used as the anticoagulant in extracorporeal haemoperfusion circuits, has now been shown to increase platelet aggregation in patients with fulminant hepatic failure and may be explained by the low circulating levels of the heparin co-factor, antithrombin III. Thus the increased platelet adhesiveness and enhanced aggregation response with heparin might both predispose to the platelet reactions during charcoal haemoperfusion. Such changes and platelet loss can be inhibited by prostacyclin infusion, making serial haemoperfusion now a routine procedure. Of the last 76 patients treated in this way, overall survival was 38% and when charcoal haemoperfusion was started in Grade III coma 65% (8).

Cirrhosis

The proportion of cirrhotic patients presenting with major clinical haemorrhage varies from centre to centre but a representative figure from one large series was 32% (9). Abnormal hepatic function in this study was more common in those who were bleeding although there was no correlation with the degree of coagulation abnormality or platelet count. The gastrointestinal tract is the major source of blood loss although the reported incidence of bleeding from variceal or non-variceal sites varies from 20% to 70% according to the hospital, degree of patient selection, frequency of alcoholism or degree of hepatic failure (Fig. 3). In a recent series of 90 patients with documented portal hypertension and oesophageal varices presenting to the Liver Unit with upper gastrointestinal bleeding, varices were the site of haemorrhage in 90% of those in whom active bleeding was observed. Although

Author	Number of patients	Oesophageal varices	Gastric varices	Other sites	Unknown	% alcoholic patients
Dagradi [1]	121	27	12	56	5	100
McCray [2]	27	19	–	74	7	100
Novis [3]	75	67	–	31	2	80
Terblanche [4]	64	72	–	28	–	NS
Waldram [5]	50	38	22	26	16	46

Figure 3. Comparison of sites of bleeding (%) in patients with oesophago-gastric varices.

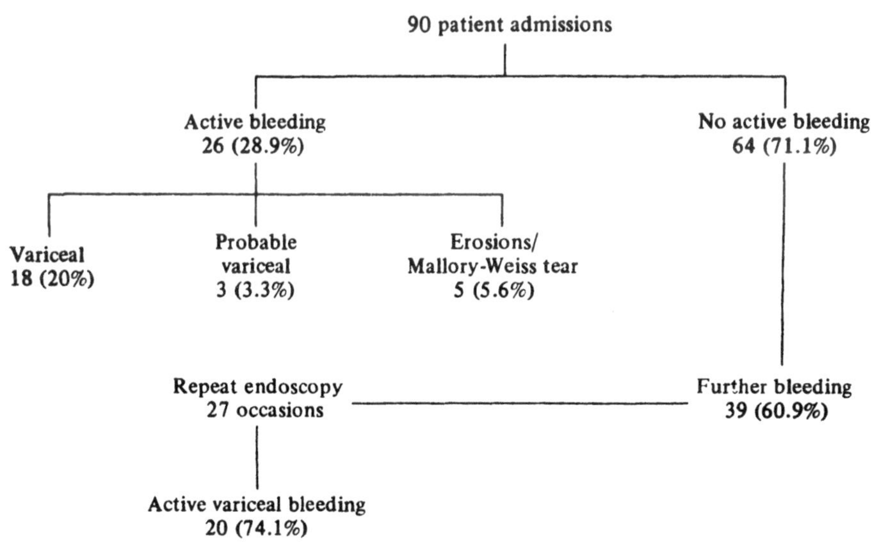

Figure 4. Endoscopy findings on 90 separate admissions and subsequent course in patients with no active bleeding at initial endoscopy.

co-existing lesions were seen in 35 cases only 5 of those (4 acute erosions and 1 Mallory Weiss tear) were the source of bleeding (Fig. 4). Varices in the region of the squamous-mucous junction of the oesophagus and stomach bled most frequently whilst bleeding from gastric varices occurred in 21% of cases. In Benhamou's study of 53 alcoholic cirrhotics with upper gastrointestinal haemorrhage, equal numbers of patients were bleeding from acute gastric erosions and oesophageal varices, although the proportion of patients with large varices was the same in both groups (10). This high frequency of haemorrhage from erosions may be related to the increased collateral circulations through the gastric and oesophageal bed which might predispose to erosive changes or increase their risk of bleeding.

The pathogenetic mechanisms underlying variceal rupture are unclear although 'erosive' and 'explosive' theories have been advanced. Gastric acid or gastro oesophageal reflux has been proposed as a cause of variceal haemorrhage from studies reporting oesophageal mucosal erosions or an increased intra-abdominal pressure due to ascites in those who have recently bled. However, there is little evidence to support such a role. Studies of oesophageal manometry, gastric acid secretion or acid clearance from the oseophagus have not revealed any abnormality in these patients (11). This is supported by the inability of cimetidine to reduce the incidence of rebleeding in patients with oesophageal varices (11) and the lack of histological evidence of oesophagitis in post mortem samples or oesphageal rings obtained during stapling transection procedures (12,13).

The explosive theory is more tenable, the size and degree of protrusion of varices, portal pressure or pressure within the varix may be responsible for bleeding. Dagradi in 1972 (14) and Palmer in 1956 (15) showed that bleeding is related to variceal size. More recently Lebrec in a series of 100 alcoholic cirrhotics admitted because of jaundice, and/or ascites, and/or gastrointestinal bleeding, showed that the prevalence of large sized oesophageal varices was much higher in those admitted with bleeding than in those with ascites or jaundice (10) (Fig. 5). Large varices are thus a risk factor for an initial bleed. Clearly portal hypertension is required for the development of varices but once present the height of the portal pressure does not appear to be a risk factor for bleeding. Reynolds (16) showed no difference in the wedged hepatic venous pressure in patients with varices with or without bleeding (Fig. 6). Several other studies have confirmed these findings (17,18).

Once a patient has bled from varices the chance of rebleeding within one year is 40% to 75%. It is important to appreciate that the factors which cause the first bleed and subsequent bleeds may be different. Westaby (19) has shown that rebleeding is nearly three times more frequent in patients with Child's Grade C liver disease than either A or B (Fig. 7). One year survival rates following bleeding with Child's Grade A and C were 75% and 30%, respectively.

In this study there was no relationship between variceal size and rebleeding, although heavy drinking and the height of the portal pressure were associated with an increased frequency of variceal haemorrhage. It is clear that in a haemodynamic system in which the activity and severity of liver disease, portal pressure, collateral flow, and variceal size are interrelated, the equation determining the risk of variceal haemorrhage is complex. The ability to identify patients at risk of bleeding is important at a time when procedures such as injection sclerotherapy and the medical treatment of portal hypertension with B-adrenergic blocking drugs are proving of value.

Figure 5. Lack of relationship between wedged hepatic vein pressure (WHVP) and bleeding from varices (from Reynolds et al).

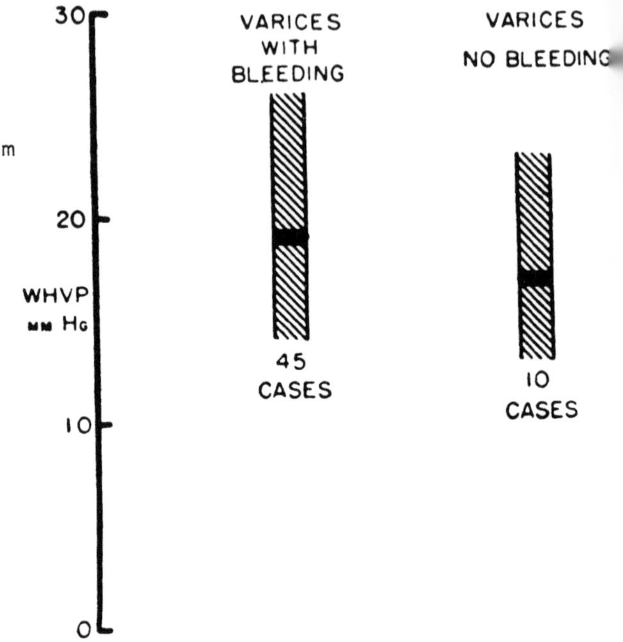

100
patients with alcoholic cirrhosis

47 admitted for ascites and/or jaundice	53 admitted for gastrointestinal bleeding

PREVALENCE OF LARGE-SIZED OESOPHAGEAL VARICES

15 (32%)	45 (85%)

$p < 0.01$

Figure 6. Prevalence of large sized oesophageal varices in patients admitted for ascites and jaundice and in patients admitted for a recent episode of gastrointestinal bledding (from Lebrec et al).

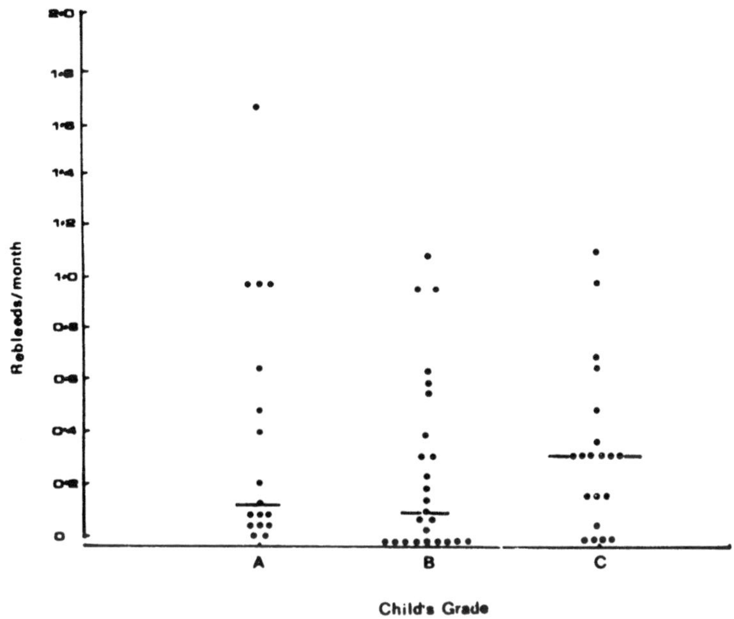

Figure 7. The relationship between the severity of the liver disease (Child's Grade) and the frequency of rebleeding (bleeds/months).

REFERENCES

1. Clark R, Rake RO, Flute PT, Williams R. 1973. Scand J Gastroenterol (Suppl) 19: 63-70
2. Williams R. 1972. Br Med Bull 28: 114-119
3. Sherlock S, Parbhoo SP. 1971. Post Grad Med J 47: 493-498
4. Gazzard BG, Portmann B, Murray-Lyon IM, Williams R. 1975. Quat J Med 176: 615-26
5. Macdougall BRD, Bailey RJ, Williams R. 1977. Lancet 1: 617-619
6. Gazzard BG, Lewis ML, Ash G, Rizz CR, Bidwell E, Williams R. 1974. Gut 15: 993-998
7. Gazzard BG, Clark R, Borirakchanyant V, Williams R. 1974. Gut 15: 88-93
8. Gimson AES, Braude S, Mellon PJ, Canalese J, Williams R. 1982. Lancet 2: 681-683
9. Spector I, Coln M. 1967. Arch Int Med 119: 577-582
10. Lebrec D, DeFleury P. Rueff B, Benhamon JP. 1980. Gastroenterology 79: 1139-114
11. Macdougall BRD, Williams R. 1983. Hepatology 1: 69-73
12. Orloff MJ, Thomas HS. 1963. Arch Surg 87: 301-307
13. Ponce J, Frouf A, De La Morena E. 1981. Hepatology 1: 641-646
14. Dagradi AE. 1972. Am J Gastroenterol 57: 520-540
15. Palmer ED, Briek IB. 1956. Gastroenterology 30: 85-90
16. Reynolds TB, Redeker AG, Geller HM. 1957. Am J Med 22: 341-350
17. Joly JG, Marlear D, Legare A. 1971. Cann Med Assoc 104: 576-580
18. Smith-Laing G, Camilo ME, Diek R, Sherlock S. 1980. Gastroenterology 78: 197-205
19. Westaby D, Macdougall BRD, Williams R. In: Variceal Bleeding. Ed. Westaby D, Macdougall BRD, Williams R. Pitman, London. 1982. p. 21-35

DISCUSSION LECTURE WILLIAMS

Question from the audience

Williams No, we would use some methadine to decrease the frequency of bleeding. If we still get gastro-intestinal bleeding in those on methadine, than we would only treat the episode of bleeding, as it occurs using whole blood. If you use plasma, there is a danger, because of the sodium that it contains and these patients are avidly retaining sodium. So we will only use fresh blood and that is when bleeding occurs.

Reding What is your opinion about the treatment of these patients with Inderal[R], do you have you any results on that?

Williams Well, our own trial at Kings' would suggest that bleeding can still occur when Inderal[R] (propanolol) is used as a prophylactic measure. We are doing a control trial in which beta-blocker is given prophylactically. Our results with propanolol are not as good with respect to prevention of further gastro-intestinal bleeding as methadine therapy, and they are not near as good as the Paris' results. They are a bit disappointing so far.

Verstraete Dr. Williams, you did expand on the pathogenesis of oesophageal bleeding in cirrhotic and non-cirrhotic patients. What is the reaction of this on giving beta-blockers in these patients?

Williams Well, beta-blockers will lower the portal pressure.

Verstraete Did I not hear you saying that there was not a good correlation between pressure and bleeding?

Williams Our results would go along with the lack of correlation that we do see in our propanolol patients, even though our studies have shown the total pressure to be reduced in those cases. But studies from other authors go strongly in favour of being a correlation.

Verstraete Well, it is remarkable that you rely more on the

results of competitive groups than on your own results. It is good to hear from the master that there is a poor correlation between patients who have bleeding and their coagulation factors; that you can find bleeding in patients with normal coagulation factors; that you can find decreased coagulation factors and no-bleeding; that you can have bleeding and correction with plasma, although your clotting factors are not necessary correct. So you are preparing for some desperate action isn't it?

Lust There are no known troubles in coagulation factors, but the conclusion on your last slide was an indication for the use of fresh blood?

Williams If somebody bleeds in cirrhosis, they have to have volume replacement anyway in hemoglobin. The conclusion of that paper from the States was that you should use fresh blood, because that was what was needed and there is no specific correlation wiht any major part of the hemostatic system. So that is why you use fresh blood, which will give you everything.

Mannucci A further comment about the absence of correlation between coagulation tests and bleeding. Some authors did biopsy with lapa roscopy; they watched the bleeding by laparoscopy coming out from the point wherever the biopsy was done. They found that the bleeding from the liver is completely independant on the values of the coaglation test, and they drew the conclusion that bleeding from biopsy was related to some hepatic abnormality

This was quite a convincing experiment and observation.

Verstraete Would you go along with the proposal that we really don't know why a patient with cirrhosis does have periodic bleedings?

Williams No, we do not know what initiates bleeding.

Verstraete And the second part is that we don't know how to treat them?

Williams Oh no, we know how to treat them. The clinicians are always better in treating than knowing why. We have good measures to treat varices now with sclerotherapy. We don't need the surgeons anymore for that.

Verstraete My question was, how to treat an existing bleeding, not to prevent bleeding?

Williams Well, the two are tied up together because there are emergency measures for stopping bleeding and the varicy of bleeding that I showed in our endoscopy study very often does stop spontaneously and clinicians, seeing a lot of varices with bleeding admitted, will know that without transfusion, their patients may actually stop bleeding for a time and than you can go on and use the injection's sclerotherapy very well.

Verstraete So they stopped bleeding spontaneously, not with standing treatment.

COAGULATION DEFECTS FOLLOWING PERITONEOVENOUS SHUNTS

D. FRANCO, C. SMADJA, A. DECORPS DECLERE

I. INTRODUCTION

Abnormal bleeding tendencies have been reported following peritoneovenous shunting of ascites in cirrhotic patients (I,I7). The eventuality of death related to diffuse bleeding in these patients has hindered the use of this procedure in such indications (8). The results of the large series recently published and of coagulation studies, have contributed to a better knowledge of the prevalence of coagulation abnormalities after peritoneovenous shunts, the type of disorders observed, their etiology and the precautions that should be undertaken to avoid severe bleeding in cirrhotic patients following such procedures.

2. NATURE OF COAGULATION DISORDERS ASSOCIATED WITH PERITONEOVENOUS SHUNT

2.I. Cirrhosis is associated with abnormalities in the coagulation process (4) which are partially explained by impaired syntheses of coagulation factors, increased destruction of platelets, increased fibrinolysis and low-grade disseminated intravascular coagulation (DIC). Following a peritoneovenous shunt, coagulation disorders described in cirrhosis worsen. There is a significant prolongation of the thrombin time, the prothrombin time and the activated partial thromboplastin time (27). A sharp decrease of the platelet count, coagulation factors V, VIII and fibrinogen is observed (I6,24,27), with an accelerated rate of fibrinogen and platelet destruction (32). Fibrinogen degradation products (FDP) are present in the blood after the operation (27). Plasma antithrombin III (AT III) decreases by 20 to 30 % (5). These changes are suggestive of DIC. In some cases fibrinolysis is associated (I).

2.2. When coagulation parameters are thoroughly studied the prevalence of DIC appears to be very high. In our series (5), DIC was evaluated in 8 cirrhotic patients using six parameters : platelet count, fibrinogen, coagulation factors V and VIII, FDP and AT III. All the patients had some variations of coagulation : two had a significant decrease of three parameters, three of 5 parameters and 3 patients of an six parameters. The onset of DIC is very rapid following an operation and reaches its peak within the first 24-48 postoperative hours (5,27). On later controls, coagulation disorders usually improve although coagulation factors and platelets often remain at lower levels than preoperatively as long as the shunt is patent (27). If the shunt is surgically interrupted or becomes obstructed, DIC disappears (I5,I6). It recurs if the shunt is re-opened or if another shunt is inserted (I6).

2.3. The prevalence of clinical bleeding in the reported series is indicated in Table I. The rate of bleeding extends over a wide range, from 2 to 37 %. Discrepancies between series might be attributed to differences in the selection of patients : a. the prevalence of clinical bleeding was the lowest in the series of Lund and Moritz (I9) who placed shunts mostly in patients with carcinomatous ascites. b. Schwartz et al (27) have pointed out that patients with a severe liver failure are most prone to bleed than others. The unusually high rate of postoperative hemorrhage in the experience of Tawes et al (32) may be related to a large number of patients with severe liver failure. Although the results of liver function tests were not given, it is stated that patients with serum bilirubin levels up to IO mg/IOO ml were included.

2.4. The severity of hemorrhagic complications varies among patients. Upper gastrointestinal bleeding may only be the consequence of portal hypertension and is not always related to coagulation defects. An ecchymosis along the subcutaneous tunnel of the venous tubing or hematomas at the site of incisions are the most frequent findings and occur in about 75 % of our patients (9). Contrariwise, the onset of diffuse bleeding is scarce (Table I), and it may occasionnally cause death, (I5, 20, 26, 27), it is an unfrequent event. A careful perusal of the literature reveals that the mortality rate ranged from 2 to 6.7 p.cent (Table I). Death from bleeding occurred mainly in patients with severe preoperative liver failure.

Table I. Coagulation disorders following peritoneovenous shunts

Authors, ref	nb of patients shunted	nb of DIC	nb of DIC related bleeding	nb of DIC related mortality
Schwartz et al (27)	I5	II (74 %)	4 (28%)	I (7 %)
Greig et al (I4)	23	9 (39 %)	I (4%)	I (4 %)
Franco et al (9)	88	88 (IOO %)	5 (6%)	2 (2 %)
Tawes et al (I3)	24	I4 (58 %)	9 (38%)	7 (29 %)
Greenlee et al (I3)	52	-	2 (4%)	2 (4 %)
Bernhoft et al (2)	5I	-	5 (IO%)	2 (4 %)
Lund and Moritz (I9)	49	-	I (2%)	I (2 %)

3. ETIOLOGY OF POST-SHUNT DIC IN CIRRHOTIC PATIENTS.

3.I. The etiology of DIC associated with peritoneovenous shunting is clearly related to the infusion of ascitic fluid in the blood of these patients. Previous experience with the Rhodiascit apparatus has shown that continuous infusion of ascites in cirrhotic patients, may lead to complications, such as a decrease of platelet count, fibrinogen and other coagulation factors and to the rise of FDP in the blood (I8,34). In one series (I8), 2.5 % of the patients treated by Rhodiascit had bleeding and one patient died of DIC. Forty-four % of the patients presented with biological signs of DIC.

3.2. It has been shown that the clotting time of normal platelet-rich plasma was shortened by the addition of ascitic fluid from a patient with postoperative DIC (24). This phenomenon might be due to the presence of procoagulant factors in the ascitic fluid. The nature of the procoagulant factors involved is not yet precisely determined. Svanberg and Astedt (3I) reported the presence of factors VII-X, V and VIII in low concentrations in the ascitic fluid and Wilkinson et al (34) also found coagulation factors in the ascitic fluid from hepatic cirrhosis. None of these levels is however sufficient to explain the shortening of the PTT of normal plasma. By studying the effect of centrifuged frozen ascitic fluids on the recalcification time of normal and heparinized plasmas and of plasmas with intrinsic factor deficiencies or deficient in factors X, VII and VII-X, Phillips and Rodgers (24) have shown that ascites acts mainly at the level of factor X. They have postulated that ascites possibly contains an already activated factor X. These findings are close to what has been described with the procoagulant properties of amniotic fluid (7, 23).

3.3. Endotoxin can promote DIC by the activation of Hageman factor (33) or by enhancing the factor X activator activity of washed human platelets (28). The combination of endotoxin and polymorphonuclear cells in the ascitic fluid could also result in the formation of a procoagulant tissue activator (2I).

However, the reality of the presence of endotoxin in ascites and blood of cirrhotic patients remains to be proven (IO). The limulus test used in most of the studies is, in effect, controversial.

4. PREDICTION OF DIC BEFORE PLACEMENT OF PERITONEOVENOUS SHUNTING.

4.I. Attempts to determine the patients which are at risk of developing DIC after a peritoneovenous shunt are quite unsuccessfull. There are very few preoperative factors which could predict the occurrence of DIC : neither plasma bilirubin levels, nor the standard coagulation tests allow to discriminate patients who will and those who will not experience DIC. Schwartz et al (27) found a significant difference in the preoperative plasma levels of factor VIII between patients who did develop (3I9%) and those who did not (III%) develop DIC after shunting. Detection of endotoxin and of FDP in ascites might indicate patients at risk of bleeding (II,25). However, the presence of endotoxin in ascites is difficult to evaluate and the presence of FDP in almost all ascites tested, renders this determination of little interest.

4.2. Bleeding occurs mainly in patients with preoperative severe liver failure (I3) and those with hepatorenal syndrom (2). A prolongation of prothrombin time to more than 6 s would identify those patients who will have a post shunt hemorrhage (I3). In our experience (9), all patients who had a preoperative plasma bilirubin level above IO mol/IOOml and plasma coagulation factors II and V, below 30 %, died postoperatively with concomitant bleeding.

5. TREATMENT OF POST SHUNT DIC

5.I. The treatment of postoperative DIC is not yet standized.

The use of heparin is controversial : in liver diseases heparin has been shown to improve coagulation but not to affect the ultimate outcome (30). After peritoneovenous shunting, heparin therapy improves thrombocytopenia and lowers plasma FDP levels (I5). The use of heparin for only a short time in all patients treated by peritoneovenous shunt is recommended by Blaisdell (3). However, the lack of scientific date showing the advantage of this treatment should restrain from its application in shunted patients.

5.2. The transfusion of platelets and fresh frozen plasma might allow to maintain the levels of fibrinogen and platelet counts above critical levels when DIC is biologically evident (I6).

5.3. Severe liver disease is associated with low AT III levels. Giles et al (I2) have shown a relationship between the pretreatment AT III levels in patients undergoing autotransfusion of concentrated ascitic fluid and the post-treatment DIC. Thus AT III infusion is expected to decrease the incidence of DIC in shunted cirrhotic patients. Boyer et al (5) found a significant reduction of DIC after 24 hours in 5 patients treated by one infusion of AT III (40 U/Kg bw) just before shunting as compared to controls shunted without AT III infusion (Table II). Furthemore there was a good correlation between the postoperative AT III levels and the intensity of DIC. This beneficial effect of AT III was not observed in a similar study of Büller and ten Cate (6) using approximately the same doses of AT III over a longer period of time. In this small series, three patients out of 5 treated by AT III did not experience DIC but the 2 others had DIC and one bled to death. The two patients who did not receive AT III had DIC. Extensive studies should be carried out on the use of AT III in cirrhotic patients treated by peritoneovenous shunt.

5.4. When severe clinical bleeding is present, interruption of the shunt usually reverses the coagulation disorders (I6). This however should be done early to avoid a fatal outcome from the general complications of DIC.

5.5. Operative removal of excessive ascitic fluid has been advocated by several authors (2,32). This lays on the assumption that the more ascitic fluid is infused, the more coagulation abnormalities occur. We have studied the effect of the intraoperative removal of 50 % of ascitic fluid at operation on the postoperative appearance of coagulation disorders (unpublished data). In 8 control patients (operated without removal of ascites), DIC was severe in 6 and moderate in 2 ; in the 8 treated patients (50 % removal of ascites at operation), DIC was absent in I and moderate in 7 (table II). Thus, removal of 50 % of the ascitic fluid during operation allows a marked and significant decrease in the importance of coagulation disorders observed after a peritoneovenous shunt in cirrhotic patients.

Table II - The effect of AT III and removal of ascitic fluid on the intensity of DIC following peritoneovenous shunt

Intensity of DIC	No treatment (8 patients)	AT III infusion (5 patients)	Removal of 50 % of ascitic fluid (8 patients)
Absent	0	3	I
Moderate	2	2	7
Severe	6	0	0

6. CONCLUSION

Peritoneovenous shunting of ascites enhances DIC in cirrhotic patients. This is due to procoagulant properties of the ascitic fluid that may lie in the presence of various procoagulant substances (activated factor X, endotoxin). Bleeding will appear when preoperative coagulation status is already disturbed (prolongation of PTT of 6 s over control, high levels of factor VIII, low levels of AT III). This may actually lead to death from diffuse bleeding in very few patients with preoperative severe liver insufficiency. The low incidence of clinical bleeding is in contrast with the high rate of coagulation disorders. The benefit of antithrombin III infusion in preventing these alterations has not yet been unequivocally demonstrated. Operative removal of ascites will decrease the intensity of coagulation defects following peritoneovenous shunt and diminish the risk of bleeding and fatal outcome. A better selection of patients, excluding those with severe liver failure should in addition make clinical bleeding an uncommon event. The coagulation disorders after peritoneovenous shunt should not therefore be an argument against this type of treatment. They represent a very interesting model for the study of DIC induction.

REFERENCES

1. Ansley JD, Bethel RA, Bowen PA, Warren WD, : Effect of peritoneovenous shunting with LeVeen valve on ascites renal function and coagulation in six patients with intractable ascites. Surgery, 1978, 83, 181-186.
2. Bernhoft RA, Pellegrini CA, Way LW : Peritoneovenous shunt for refractory ascites. Arch Surg, 1982, 117, 631-635.
3. Blaisdell FW : Discussion of Tawes RL, Sydorak GR, Kennedy PA, Brown WH, Scribner RG, Beare JP, Harros EJ : Coagulopathy associated with peritoneous shunting. Am J. surg, 1981, 142, 51-55.
4. Bloom AL : Intravascular coagulation and the liver. Br. J. Hematol, 1975, 30, 1-7.
5. Boyer C, Wolf M, Lavergne JM, Haiat A, Descorps Declère A, Franco D, Larrieu MJ : Prevention of disseminated intravascular coagulation after LeVeen peritoneovenous shunts by infusion of AT III concentrates. Sixth International Congress on Thrombosis of the Mediterranean League against Thromboembolic Disease, Monte-Carlo Oct 23-25, 1980, Abst 218.
6. Büller HR, Ten Cate JW : Antithrombin III infusion in patients undergoing peritoneovenous shunt operation :

failure in the prevention of disseminated intravascular coagulation. In Büller HR : Studies on antithrombin III and human antithrombin III concentrate transfusion. Rodopic, Amsterdam, I98I, I45-I68.

7. Courtney LD, Allington M : Effect of amniotic fluid on blood coagulation. Br J Hematol, I972, 22, 353-355.
8. Epstein M : Peritoneovenous shunt in the management of ascites and hepatorenal syndrome. Gastroenterology, 82, 790-799.
9. Franco D, Cortesse A, Castro e Sousa F, Bismuth H : Dérivation péritonéo-jugulaire dans le traitement de l'ascite irréductible du cirrhotique : résultats chez 88 malades. Gastroentérol Clin Biol, I98I, 5, 393-402.
IO. Fulenwider JT, Sibley C, Stein SF, Evatt B, Nordlinger BM, Ivey GL : Endotoxemia of cirrhosis : an observation not substantiated. Gastroenterology, I980, 78, IOOI-IOO4.
II. Fumarola D : Coagulopathy following peritoneovenous shunting - an endotoxin mediation ? Surgery, I980, 87, 475.
I2. Giles AR, Sauder D, Seaton TL, Johnston M, Hirsh J : Changes in the coagulation status of patients undergoing autotransfusion of concentrated ascitic fluid as treatment of refractory ascites. Blood, I977, 50 (suppl), 267 (abst).
I3. Greenlee HB, Stanley MM, Reinhardt GD : Intractable ascites treated with peritoneovenous shunts (LeVeen). Arch Surg, I98I, II6, 5I8-524.
I4. Greig PD, Langer B, Blendis LM, Taylor BR, Glym MFX : Complications after peritoneovenous shunting for ascites. Am. J. Surg, I980, I39, I25-I3I.
I5. Harmon DC, Demirjian Z, Ellman L, Fisher JE : Disseminated intravascular coagulation with the peritoneovenous shunt. Ann Int Med I979, 90, 774-776.
I6. Lerner RG, Nelson JC, Corines P, del Guercio LRM : Disseminated intra-vascular coagulation. Jama, I978, 240, 2064-2066.
I7. LeVeen HH, Wapnick S, Grosberg S, Kinney MJ : Further experience with peritoneovenous shunt for ascites. Ann Surg, I976, I84, 574-58I.
I8. Levy VG, Pouleau N, Opolon P, Caroli J : Treatment of ascites by reinfusion of concentrated peritoneal fluid. Post-Grad Med J, I975, 5I, 564-566.
I9. Lund RH, Moritz MW : Complications of Denver peritoneovenous shunting. Arch Surg I982, II7, 924-928.
20. Matseshe JW, Beart RW, Bartholomew LG, Baldus WP : Fatal disseminated intravascular coagulation after peritoneovenous shunt for intractable ascites. Mayo Clin Proc I978, 53, 526-528.
2I. Niemitz J, Monisan DC : Lipid A ast he biologically active moiety in bacterial endotoxin (LPS) - initiated generation of prociagulant activity by peripheral blood leukocytes. Blood I977, 49, 947-95I.
22. Paliard P, Partensky C, Sauvier E : Ascite irréductible

cirrhotique. Résultats de la dérivation péritonéo-jugulaire chez I6 malades. Nouv. Presse Méd., I98I, IO, 27I5-27I8.

23. Phillips LL, Davidson EC : Procoagulant properties of amniotic fluid. Am J Obstet Gynecol I972, II3, 9II-9I9.
24. Phillips LL, Rodgers JB : Procoagulant activity of ascitic fluid in hepatic cirrhosis. In vivo and in vitro. Surgery, I979, 86, 7I4-72I.
25. Puig JG, Anton FM, Gonzalez JM, Vazquez JO : Peritoneovenous shunt and bacterial endotoxin. Mayo Clin Proc, I979, 54, I33 (letter).
26. Robert A, Bloch P, Boinot C, Lévy VG, Huguet C : Coagulopathie de consommation après dérivation péritonéo-jugulaire. Gastroentérol Clin Biol, I980, 4, 389.
27. Schwartz ML, Swaim WR, Vogel SB : Coagulopathy following peritoneovenous shunting. Surgery, I979, 85, 67I-676.
28. Semeraro N, Fumarola D, Mertens F, Vermylen J : Evidence that endotoxins enhance the factor X activator of washed human platelets. Br J Hematol, I978, 38, 243-249.
29. Stein SF, Fulenwider JT, Ansley JD : Accelerated fibrinogen and platelet destruction after peritoneovenous shunting (LeVeen valve implantation). Gastroenterology, I978, 74, II6I (abst).
30. Straub PW : Diffuse intravascular coagulation in liver disease ? Semin Thromb Hemostasis, I977, 4, 29-39.
3I. Svanberg L, Astedt B : Coagulative and fibrinolytic properties of ascitic fluid associated with ovarian tumors. Cancer, I975, 35, I382-I387.
32. Tawes RL, Sydorak GR , Kennedy PA, Brown WH, Scribner RG, Beare JP, Harris EJ : Coagulopathy associated with peritoneovenous shunting. Am J Surg, I98I, I42, 5I-55.
33. Wilkinson SP, Arroyo T, Gazzaid BG, Moodie H, Williams R : Relation of renal impairment and hemorrhagic diathesis to endotoxoemia in fulminant hepatic failure. Lancet, I974, I, 52I-524.
34. Wilkinson SP, Davidson AR, Henderson J, Williams R : Ascites reinfusion using the Rhodiascit apparatus clinical experience and coagulation abnormalities. Postgrad Med J, I975, 5I, 583-585.

DISCUSSION LECTURE FRANCO

Williams	Could you comment the use of steroids directly into the ascitic fluid?
Franco	I've heard it, but I did not read this paper.
Williams	It was supposed to turn off fibrinolytic activation.
Baele	I would like to add something. About three years ago an American group reported in the American Journal of Haematology that the collagen is present in ascitic fluid and may be activation of the platelets and also the clotting system.
Franco	Thank you for your information, I do think there are plenty of activators in ascitic fluid. We don't know yet that is the reason in which DIC is constant in those patients.
De Groote	Occlusion of the shunt could be related to the material you use.
Franco	Yes I think it is a good remark. We have a twenty percent rate of late occlusion or obstruction of the shunt and we've tried to determine if this was related to the severity of post-operative D.I.C. We could not demonstrate it. What I think is that thrombosis is related to the kind of material we use, and we recently changed the venous tubing of the shunt and we decreased very much the incidence of thrombosis. I think we can improve the results of the shunt using different kind of material.
Verstraete	Could you define what you mean by "late" occlusion of the shunt, what is "late" in terms of days or weeks?
Franco	Usually thrombosis occurs at about between 2 or 6 months. In our experience, it is almost always after 2 months but sometimes, in 2 patients, we've observed very early thrombosis. In one of these patients AT III was very low and perhaps this was related to the early thrombosis.
Ten Cate	I am well aware of your data and I'll try to under-

stand the difference between your and our study results. But I understood that you have a moderate beneficial effect of one bolus injection of human AT-III concentrate in the prevention of D.I.C. My questions are: -Are you still using AT III concentrate to prevent DIC in such patients? I may understand that initial D.I.C., occuring in the first days following surgery, may be prevented by removal of ascites in the preoperative phase and secondly by the administration of AT III concentrate. However, in the follow-up of these patients, severe D.I.C. with low fibrinogen levels may be observed at days 4, 5 , 6, 7 postoperatively. Do you prevent D.I.C. in this later stage following surgery?

Franco First of all, we don't use anymore AT III for one main reason: it is very expensive to get it. I think it was very interesting to choose the effect. We don't do it anymore because we didn't remove ascites when we used AT III. We used to remove about 10 percent of ascites in the control blood and in the AT III treated group. Later on we removed 50 percent of ascites and we found that this decreased the severity of D.I.C., so we didn't use anymore the AT III concentrate. I showed on the first slide that the coagulation disorders after the shunt are at the highest level on the first and second postoperative days in our experience. And that is why if you go through this initial period, you still have some coagulation disorders later. You can have a fibrinogen level below 1 gram per liter, but we've never, in our experience, observed a worsening of D.I.C. on the 6th or 7th postoperative day. I wonder if the reports of secondary D.I.C. are not related to septicemia for example.

Verstraete Are you satisfied dr. Ten Cate?

Ten Cate Our observations clearly indicate ongoing D.I.C. from the first postoperative days onwards, and is certainly observed at around the 5th until the 7th day. Continuous infusion of ascites may in part explain this phenomenon.

Franco If you tell the patients 6 months later they still hav D.I.C., but low grade D.I.C., that is very important. And I don't think there is any harm to get some D.I.C. in a longer period.

Baele Have you looked at the AT III level?

Franco We have looked and measured AT III in plasma and we found that the lowest AT III was after the operation, the greatest D.I.C. we've obtained.

Verstraete Would it be sensible to infuse continuously mini doses of heparin with a slower release of the micro-injector in the peritoneal fluid?

Franco This has been recommended by one or two people, and we do it for the last 20 patients, but not to prevent D.I. but to try to avoid thrombosis, because I think thromb sis starts evidently late. We give subcutaneous low dos of subcutaneous heparin on which we have no harmful effect with this treatment. I hope we will have less thrombosis.

Verstrate My idea, a very naïve idea, is not to give it subcutane ly, but to give it intra the peritorium. I mean on the spot with a micro processor. Ways today is to give very small minor doses, there where you want to give it, jus to avoid the generalization of the effect of heparin th you would have limited to there where you want to have it.

Franco I think, when you put a valve in a cirrhotic patient, you get the first infectious risk and I would not like to put a second risk of infection in one cirrhotic patient by adding a pump.

BLEEDING DURING ORTHOTOPIC LIVER TRANSPLANTATION IN MAN

G.W. van Imhoff, H. Wesenhagen, E. Haagsma, C.Th. Smit Sibinga, R.A.F. Krom and C.H. Gips

Severe non surgical bleeding has grave implications for the outcome of orthotopic liver transplantation (OLT) in man. Pathological fibrinolysis and consumption coagulopathy (1-5) have both been implicated. The use of E aminocapronic acid (E.A.C.A.) led to severe thromboembolic complications in man, and bleeding was not always prevented (1,2). Further, in dogs, neither E.A.C.A. nor heparin could influence changes in coagulation and fibrinolysis during OLT (3), while in man severe bleeding was seen from even small amounts of heparin (5). Both in animals and in men changes seemed related to the quality of the donor liver (2,3,5).

However, in our series of OLT, no difference could be found in the quality of graft, measured by donor age, cause of death; ischaemia times, preservation technique, early biochemistry and histology, between early survivors (> 7 days) and non survivors (< 7 days). But patients with severe bloodloss (> 6 liter) during OLT had impaired survival compaired to patients with relatively normal bloodloss (< 6 L). Parameters of coagulation and fibrinolysis were studied prospectively before and on fixed times during OLT, while using a standard transfusion protocol in 11 consecutive recipients (OLT 10-20) to answer the following questions.

Can severe bloodloss be predicted before OLT and/or can it be explained from the course of parameters during OLT?

Methods

Studied parameters were, prothrombin time (PT), activated partial thromboplastin time (APTT), reptilasetime (RT), factors I-XII, antithrombin III activity (AT III), plasminogen activity, α2 antiplasmin activity (α 2 AP) and fibrin (ogen) degradation products (F.D.P.) as well as platelet counts. The standard transfusion protocol contained fresh frozen plasma (1.5 - 3 U/hr) cryoprecipiate (2-4 U/hr) and platelet concentrates. Red blood cells with or without cryosupernatant plasma depending on volume need were given to compensate for bloodloss.

Results

1) Bloodloss

Severe non surgical bleeding characterized by diffuse oozing was encountered in three patients (OLT 13,18,20). In OLT 13 (bloodloss 14 liter) bleeding could be managed. In OLT 18 (bloodloss 42 liter) bleeding finally stopped after 9 hours. In OLT 20 (bloodloss 45 liter) bleeding could not be managed and the patient finally exsanguinated in the operating theatre. Bloodloss in the other 8 patients was less than 6 liter and no haemostatic problems were encountered.

Severe bleeding did not seem to be influenced by transfusion of FFP, cryoprecipitate and platelets nor by tranexaminic acid (OLT 18, 20) and PPBS (OLT 20) administered in the recirculation phase when severe bleeding had already occurred.

Bloodloss in OLT 13,18 and 20 was already severe and markedly different from the other patients before recirculation.

2) Parameters of coagulation and fibrinolysis

Low pre-operative values of FII, FVII, FIX, AT III ($p < 0{,}01$) and FI, FX, α 2 AP ($p < 0.025$) as well as prolonged P.T. ($p < 0.025$) correlated with total bloodloss during OLT.

However individual patients with severe bleeding (> 6 L) could not be separated from those with normal bloodloss (< 6 L) on the basis of these parameters.

During operation while using the transfusion protocol a specific pattern of changes in parameters could be seen in all patients. A significant decrease especially one hour after recirculation of FVIII-C, FV and FX, a rise of FDP in the anhepatic phase and after recirculation and a moderate but consistent decrease in α2 AP was seen. There was no significant change in the other parameters studied. Although consistent with consumption coagulopathy, interpretation of these results is hazardous because, even in those patients without apparent haemostatic problems, total bloodloss and transfusion often equalled the bloodvolume of the recipient.
No consistent difference could be found in the course or absolute values of parameters studied between patients with severe bloodloss and the others. In none of the three patients with severe bleeding a specific diagnosis as to the cause of non surgical bleeding could be made clinically or in the laboratory.

Conclusions:

1. Total bloodloss during OLT is correlated with pre-operative coagulation and fibrinolysis parameters.
2. Excessive bleeding is already heralded before recirculatic

Thus: recipient factors play a major role in OLT outcome.

3. When during OLT excessive bleeding occurs it is very difficult to influence.
4. Excessive bleeding can not be explained from the results of the coagulation and fibrinolysis tests during OLT.

Unfortunately, excessive bleeding remains an important and unsolved problem in human livertransplantation.

REFERENCES

1. Von Kaulla KN, Kaye H, von Kaulla E, Marchioro TL, Starzl TE. Changes in blood coagulation. Arch. Surg. 92: 71-79, 1966.
2. Groth CG, Pechet L, Starzl TE. Coagulation during and after orthotopic transplantation of the human liver. Arch. Surg. 98: 31-34, 1969.
3. Pechet L, Groth CG, Daloze PM. Changes in coagulation and fibrinolysis after orthotopic canine liver homotransplantation. J. Lab. Clin. Med. 73: 91-102, 1969.
4. Flute PT, Rake MO, Williams R, Seaman MJ, Calne RY. Livertransplantation in man -IV, haemorrhage and thrombosis. Br. Med. J. 3: 20-23, 1969.
5. Bohmig HJ. The coagulation disorder of orthotopic hepatic transplantation. Sem. Thromb. and Haemost. 4: 57-82, 1977.

DISCUSSION LECTURE VAN IMHOFF

Williams I am very interested to see the results. I would agree with you entirely that once severe bleeding occurs, you can't correct them. But I think there is one point you did not stress sufficiently or you did not consider, and that is the extent of the surgical section of collateral channels in the cirrhotic patients with severe portal hypertension. And I don't know how many of those you have in your series. One of the important factors, I think, is the amount of the section.

Van Imhoff I think you are right. We analyzed the duration of the unhepatic phase in our patients and we could find no significantly differences between those patients who lacked and those patients who didn't. On the other hand, we noticed that patients who bled extensively, all fall into the group of patients with chronic acitive cirrhosis and not in the patients within the group of primary biliary cirrhosis. This could of course mean that we have not done enough transplantations yet in the PBC group and we should wait and see what happens when we'll have to transplant severely ill PBC patients. Maybe we'll get him in a better condition. I think the number of patients is insufficient to make any analysis on the basis of the extent of the surgical procedure at this moment.

Mannucci You showed a group of patients with cirrhosis and with very high or normal levels of coagulation factors. Are these patients having other special features?

Van Imhoff We find normal or even high levels of all clotting factors. Only factor V sometimes is dropping below the line of 50 percent. This is something we noticed, yes. We probably get them earlier, because this is the type of patient who is in bed and not walking around while synthesis functions of the liver is not too bad.

Giddings After the addition of dropping clotting factor activity especially related to factor V an VIII, they are very well stabilized, but all those factors considered adequate, could not be adequate for haemostasis. I always believed that this level is much higher than that in haemofilia..

Van Imhoff I would like to answer in two parts. You are right. I don't know, it is very difficult to say anything about really hemostatic safe levels of these factors together because we only know something about the congenital deficiencies. There are some papers about: what is hemostatically safe? Mostly it is about 30 - 40 percent. On the other hand, we could find no differences in the absolute values, or in the changes of parameters during the operation between those patients who bled severely and those patients who didn't have any hemostatic problem during the operation. I can come back to what Prof. Williams said during his talk: it seems to be not the coagulation factors, but the initial situation what the thing that happens and what starts the bleeding. Then when you are low, you are getting to problems.

Giddings I was thinking more in terms of your 40 percent being inadequate really, and most haemofiliacs, anyway, are bleeding subsequent the surgery. So that the level at that time is really not important for the surgical bleeding, but maybe subsequentally important and I believe dr. Mannucci will tell us what he feels about levels being higher than that in serious surgery.

Van Imhoff I don't think you can compare this kind of patients with hemophilia.

MAIN PROBLEMS IN THE TREATMENT OF BLEEDING IN CIRRHOTIC PATIENTS

POTRON G. , DROULLE C. , N'GUYEN P. , ADJIZIAN J.C. , POYNARD A. , LEHN E. , LIRZON P. , PIGNON B. , ETIENNE J.C.

Haemorrhagic disorders are intricated in patients with liver cirrhosis. The vascular phenomen and the abnormalities of the digestive tract are, at least, as important as the hemostasis pattern disorders ; which need not only to be substituted but must also be treated in physiological ways. This implies a rather difficult diagnostic approach but at the same time it allows the resolution of the different problems.

1. THE DEFECT IN SYNTHESIS OF COAGULATION FACTORS.

A low level of the coagulation factors in plasma does not always prove a deficient synthesis. However, a parallel decrease in both functionnal and antigenic activities allows a diagnostic approach (35). Conventionnally, this defect concerns VII, V, X, II, IX factors ; meanwhile, there is also a fall in fibrinogen and in factor XIII.

The treatment of such defects in production is mainly substitutive but it also supposes several problems :

1.1 Indications for the treatment :

A haemorrhagic syndrom is rarely due, to the fall of each factor but rather occurs in the case of other disfunctions.
The analysis of "the factors of risks" forms the subject of another paper (SAMAMA). However, let us remark that there is a defect, in both activator and inhibitor factors in cirrhotic patients. Antithrombin III (AT III) is very low in these patients (32) and the antithrombin III rate per coagulation factors seems to be a good index of the risks encountered by the patients (4, 32, 48). A positive ratio (antithrombin III level lower than coagulation factors), is an index of hypercoagulability

rather than an index of hypocoagulability; phlebitis, pulmonary embolism, portal thrombosis, are not unusual in such patients. A negative ratio indicated a risk of haemorrhagic complication (fig. 1):

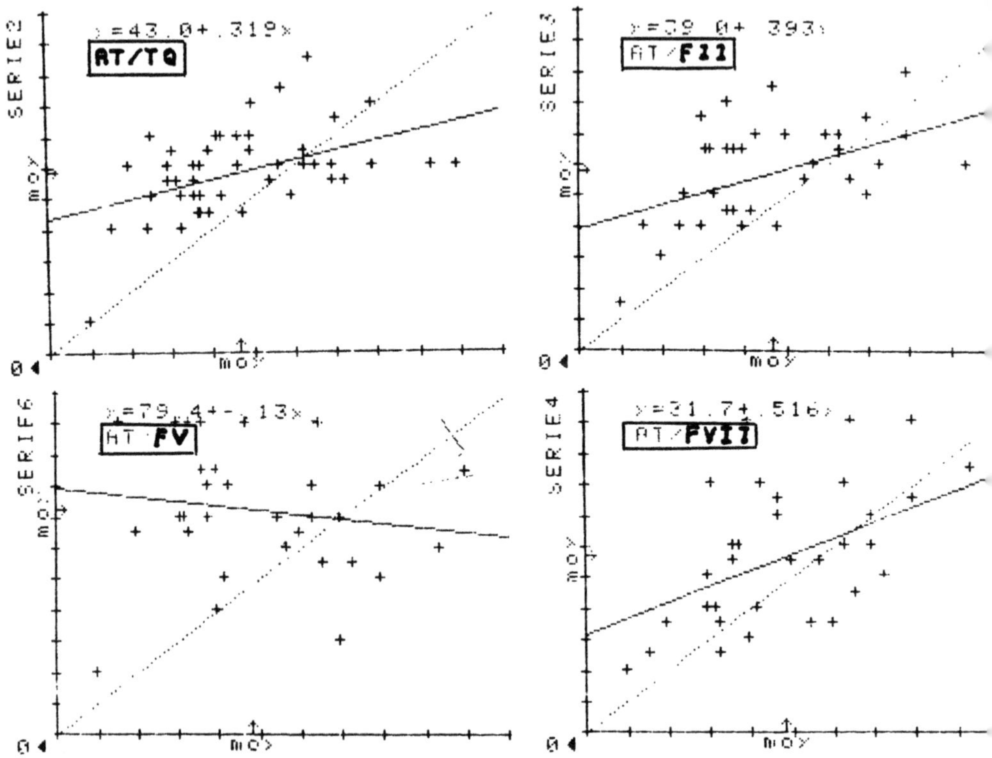

Fig. 1 : Correlation between antithrombin III and coagulation factors in 18 patients with liver cirrhosis.

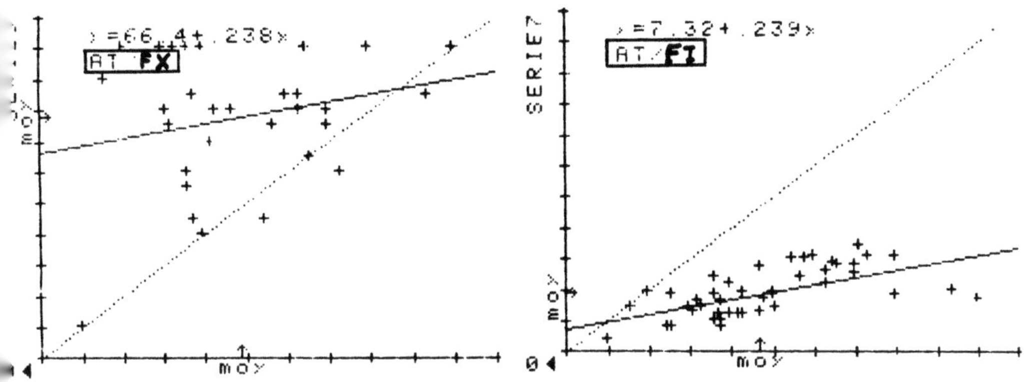

Fig. 1 : Correlation between antithrombin III and coagulation factors in 18 patients with liver cirrhosis.

An α_2 macroglobulin high rate and an α_1 antitrypsin normal rate is, according to some authors, a physiological means to restore the balance (13). This notion requires a better knowledge of the physiological participation of these molecules in vivo.

In the case of digestive bleeding, the problem is much more important. Substitution seems to be logical in order to assure, at least during several days, a satisfactory hemostasis, allowing a possible local treatment. As to minor operation or even an hepatic biopsy, only if the defect is important, substitution is required in order to correct temporarily in the synthesis defect.

1.2 <u>Choice of substitution products</u> :

Because of the new chromatographic method, french "PPSB" and some "Prothrombin Complex" have grown poorer in factor VII (14), therefore compensation is very incomplete, factor VII has the shortest life. However, some of these unbalanced products contain activated factors (89) and when injected in patients with weak inhibitors capacity, they can lead to disseminated intravascular coagulation (D.I.C.), fibrinolysis or thrombosis (8,15,44,57,58,89).

Some products, such as Proplex (Fenwall), have sucessfully used ind the correction of Quick time, without starting DIC.
Prothromplex (Immuno) can give quite satisfactory results without any signs of coagulopathy, if associated with factor VII.

Some authors have even suggested a substitution of factor VII before hepatic biopsy, in order to prevent coagulopathy after Prothrombin Complex substitution (37). Such methods must be carefully used and the lack of activated factors must be previously determined for each lot/

Fresh frozen plasma is the only balanced product (table 1)

	CONGELATION		
	Before (n=20)	6 weeks (n=20)	12 weeks (n=10)
Fibrinogen	3,22 ± 0,59	2,34 ± 0,65	-
Factor II (%)	91 ± 9	92 ± 8	96 ± 4
Factor VII (%)	79 ± 12	76 ± 16	75 ± 12
Factor X (%)	92 ± 10	90 ± 10	92 ± 11
Factor V (%)	90 ± 9	92 ± 9	-
Factor VIII (%)	97 ± 21	48 ± 22	Willebrand 80 to 90
Thrombin time (%)	20,1 ± 2,0	19,4± 1,8	19,0 ± 4,2
Bothrops time (%)	19,3 ± 1,9	20,1 ± 2,2	20,7 ± 5,8
Plg (%)	93 ± 13	95 ± 15	92 ± 12
FDP (g/1)	-	-	-
Gelation test	2+	0+	0+
ATIII (%)	100 ± 30	105 ± 34	106 ± 38

Table 1 : The different coagulation parameters of fresh plasma before and after preservation at -80° C.

Since the concentration of coagulation factors and of inhibitors is equal, its only defect is to require large volumes and to bring other proteins and sodium. The risk of B hepatitis transmission is reduced, thanks to satisfactory case findings but the problem of non A and non B hepatitis is not yet resolved. However, its preparation requires some precautions: a quick separation of plasma after collection, an important centrifugation, to obtain a plasma poor in platelets (< 30.10^9/liter), conservation at -40° C or better at -80° C, a quick thawing and warming at 30°C to render cryofibrinogen soluble.

All these products are indicated for short periods only, for example, surgical interventions or hepatic biopsy. They can be stopped before healing when local haemostasis is satisfactory in patients with no other particular abnormalities in their fibrinolytic system. The efficiency is always brief so a subsitution has to be made again (83). In the case of overload a substitution of prothrombin complex associated with fresh plasma can be used. Thus, the risk of thrombosis is reduced due to the dilution of the activated factors (56).

2. PRESENCE OF ABNORMAL MOLECULES.

They are mainly dysfibrinogenemia, found in cirrhosis as well as in hepatitis or in hepatic metastasis. The analysis has been the subject of many studies, but here 3 problems avise (1,20,29,65,82) :

2.1. Is there any haemorrhagic risk ?

A categorical answer is difficult. However, monomers polymerisation disorder can certainly be responsible for a distant bleeding relapse and formed thrombus, particularly sensitive to plasmin, especially in case of a defect in factor XIII.

Fresh frozen plasma substitution does not always improve the coagulation times (in vitro); moreover an imperfect freezing leads to fibrin monomers polymersisation disorders. However, the substitution of fibrinogen concentrates (in which the molecules are particularly damaged during the preparation) and/or even of cryoprecipitates, are not justified but the latter has the advantage of adding factor XIII.

2.2. What is the prognostic value ?

Among 500 patients with hepatic disease, we have reported 93 abnormalities in the fibrinogen polymerisation. 3 stages were established according to the curve of polymerisation and on the evolution of the disturbance in the plasma during its conservation. The fibrinogen lesion is important more especially as the hepatic disorder is severe (table 2). The clinical and biological aggravation always appears with a worsening of the fibrinogen lesion

	N	A	B	C
Group I (alcoholic polynevritis)	10	100		
Group II (stabilited cirrhosis)	3	37	67	0
Group III (icteroascitic)	41	12	52	36
Group IV (bleeding)	6	16	51	53
Group V (coma)	8	0	25	75

Table 2 : Correlations between fibrinogen polymerisation abnormalities and the importance of hepatic disorder (alcohol intoxication) (A,B,C are expressed in %).

2.3. Effects on the biological tests

Abnormal molecules lead to a prolongation of the thrombin and the reptilase times. The results of fibrinogen determination vary with the method used (low by Von Clauss, normal by heat precipitation or immunology). Their association with the marks of the defect in synthesis can give a wrong picture of consommation coagulopathy. The systematic use of 2 techniques of fibrinogen determination by the thrombin time, with an increasing concentration of thrombin and even by the fibrinogen polymerisation curve, allows diagnosis.

3. CONSUMPTION COAGULOPATHY

The existence of consumption coagulopathy is determined by biological tests (12, 39, 85, 91, 93), increase of fibrinogen or prothrombin turnover (11, 22, 23, 28) and with the efficiency of heparinotherapy (22, 33, 43, 86, 94, 99). However, biological demonstrations remain quite difficult. The decrease in factors, depends partly on a defect in synthesis; thrombocytopenia is also linked to a splenic sequestration. The presence of fibrin degradation products can be seen in dysfibrinogenemia or fibrinolysis (chap. 4). The determination of fibrin soluble complex (18) and particularly of fibrinopeptide A is of great contribution in the absence of thrombotic disease. The coagulopathy mechanism is not well known, but promotes specific problems in cirrhotic patients, thus, so they always require an adequate therapy.

3.1. The excess of activators.

They may be provided by cellular lysis, more particularly in hepatitis. However, hemolysis is not rare (36,50). In this particularly unstable system (low rate of factors and also of inhibitors) activators can lead to a coagulopathy (even when they have no visible effect in a normal patient).

The activity of these activators is increased by the lack of clearance of activators and of activated factors. Also the diffusion of endotoxins from the bowel through the portal system leads to a triggering of the haemostatic system (56).

3.2. The lack of inhibitors undoubtely plays a very important part.

The low rate of antithrombin III can hardly stop intravascular coagulation.

3.3 The defect in plasminogen can favour the deposits of fibrin. This can lead to an alteration of the function of some organs and especially of liver. The rather low rate of fibrin degradation products does not increase the hypocoagulability.

3.4. Stasis in the portal system, the collateral circulation and more over in the splenic circulation increases the phenomen of splenic sequestration (38). Indeed, splenectomy leads to an increase of factors V, VII and X and of platelets (53,92).

This coagulopathy is characterized by a chronic and rather stable evolution. However, any abnormal stimulation of coagulation such as PPSB or even preserved blood (with activated factors) can lead to an haemorragic syndrom. Such is the case of the erythrocyte concentrates where 30 % of the residual plasma is rich in thromboplastin, phospholipids and so on. Such patients should only receive erythrocyte concentrates which are washed or preserved for less than eight days. Heparin appears to be a logical therapeutic agent against the activation by activators. Some authors state such assays with success (21,23,33,42, 74,99). The heparinotherapy must be rigorously achieved :

3.4.1 Subcutaneous administration has to be carefully used in patients with an important thrombocytopenia, a low rate of coagulation factors and with an increased vascular fragility. They can only be used after the most important abnormalities have been corrected.

3.4.2 It is quite difficult to determine the dosage. It seems logical to start the treatment with a small posology. Thrombocytopenia and the low rate of the hemostatic system can lead to an important bleeding tendency if the anticoagulant effect is too high. In litterature, the doses stated vary from 12.000 U.I (21,74,99) to 50.000 (90). We used mainly doses of 15.000 U.I. calcium heparinate daily from 15 days to 3 months.

3.4.3 Surveillance is one of the most difficult tasks : although they are generally long at the beginning, the activated cephalin time and the thrombin time (compared to the reptilase time) are the main tests. The mesurement of heparinotherapy cannot be performed on the basis of the calibration of these tests, which are not abnormal before any treatment. The chromogenic substrate test (anti-Xa or anti-IIa effect) remain questionnable. The defect in antithrombin III explains that the results may be different whether the reagent brings antithrombin III or not (fig.2). However, the difference in the inhibiting activities after an administration of antithrombin III in vitro, will signal to the clinician that substitution rich in antithrombin III may lead to a very important hypocoagulability. In the same way, in vitro addition of heparin in cirrhotic plasma, gives weak hypocoagulability (fig. 3). This abnormality is not totally reversible by means of the in vitro antithrombin III addition. The heparin neutralising activity of the plasma is increased in patients with liver cirrhosis.

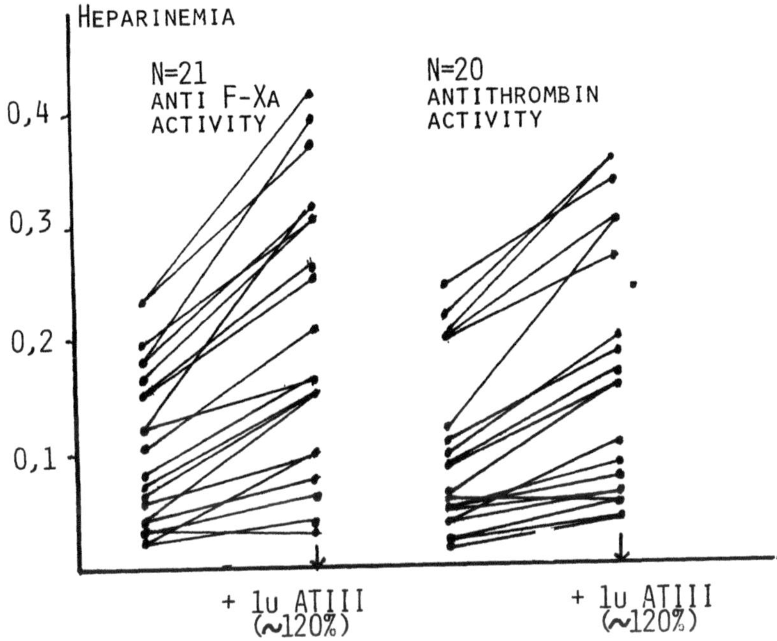

Fig. 2 : Antithrombin III values in the pathologic plasma : 20-40 %
(chromogenic substrate assay - Kem-O-Mat Coultronics, chromothrombin F Xa Stago, S 2338 thrombin -Kabi without and with in vitro Antithrombin III addition).

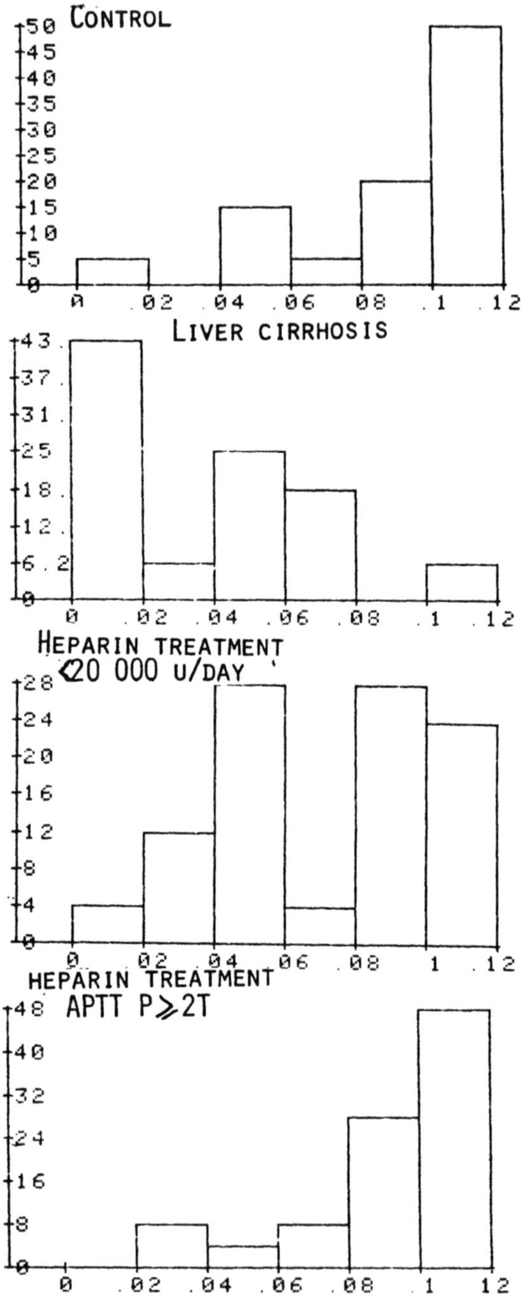

Fig. 3:Heparin neutralising activity of plasma in patients with liver cirrhosis or during heparin therapy. Variations of APTT.

The reduction of the hyperdestruction of fibrinogen or platelets cannot be easily made. The disappearance of fibrinopeptid A is undoubtedly one of the most reliable index but this determination is not yet commonly made (18). The disappearance of high molecular weight fibrinogen is much more difficult to determine and seems to be dissociated from fibrinopeptid A, as if it constituted a different physiological element. The normalisation of B thromboglobulin can be an interesting parameter but it is correlated with a more complex phenomen.

3.4.4 Some authors suggested a substitution of fresh frozen plasma in association with heparinotherapy to prevent any risk of hypocoagulability. This attitude is not required to reduce the phenomen of coagulopathy with small heparin dosis.

On the contrary, blood transfusion in cirrhotic patients with disseminated intravascular coagulation needs a treatment with heparin as it brings activated factors. We notice 2 different results after heparinotherapy. A good clinical improvement is correlated to a good improvement of the different biological paramenters. However, there is not correction of the biological tests in patients with a bad clinical evolution. The way it has been applied (constant doses of 15.000 I.U. daily, calcium heparinate), treatment with heparin is inconstantly efficient. (table 3)

	Favorable n=17		Defavorable n=15	
	before	after	before	after
Quick (%)	51±22	63±19	44±11	43±16
II (%)	47±15	59±17	44±13	40±14
II Taipan%	65±20	62±24	43±4	37±14
II Staphy%	38±25	53±32	35±14	28±9
V (%)	65±27	74±22	51±23	49±17
VII+X (%)	36±21	54±22	35±18	29±14
Plg(%)	47±16	67±23	39±18	45±21
Fibrinogen g/l	2,5±1,3	3,16±1	2,6±1,1	2,45±0,85
Platelets $10^3/\mu l$	122±73	162±95	108±81	105±99

Table 3 : Variations in plasmatic coagulation factors after treatment by heparin (favorable and unfavorable are clinical results).

Antithrombin III substitution is quite recent and a logical discovery. It normalizes the increased fibrinogen turn over (79).
The lack of inhibitors is particularly obvious when ascitis liquid is intravascularlt transfered through Le Veen shunts.
Ascitis is rich in inhibitors and activators and therefore important coagulopathy occurs (table 4).

ASCITIS n=12		
1) Transfers (APTT)		
	normal plasma	patient plasma
anticoagulant	7	10
activation	2	0
no effect	3	2
2) Fibrinogen degradation products		
>80 ug/ml	2	
20<<80 ug/ml	3	
<20 ug/ml	7	
3) Antithrombin III	$10,2\pm8\%$	
plasminogen	$4,2\pm3\%$	
α_2 fast antiplasmin	$12,1\pm7,4\%$	
prekallikrein	$1,4\pm1,5\%$	
fibrinogen <0,4 g/l=11		
1,4 g/l=1 (after other ponction)		

Table 4 : Coagulation parameters of ascitis from 12 patients with liver cirrhosis.

4. ABNORMALITIES OF FIBRINOLYSIS.

Hyperfibrinolysis is often refered to occur during hepatic cirrhosis. Several mechanisms have been advocated, each of which requires specific treatment.

4.1 Excess of circulating activators.

This rather old hypothesis is not always easy to demonstrate because of the difficulty to interprete the euglobulin lysis test in cirrhotic patients. The lack of clearance of the activators (34) and the vascular anomalies can sometimes explain their increase. It is worth noticing the great sensibility of these patients to such products as nicotinic acid (46,76,96) or catecholamines (27,45). The normal "tolerance" phenomen to the repetition of injections is not found but such a sensibility seems to be bound to plasmatic lack of balance.

4.2 Lack of balance of the fibrinolytic system

The circulating plasminogen level is low (fig. 4) :

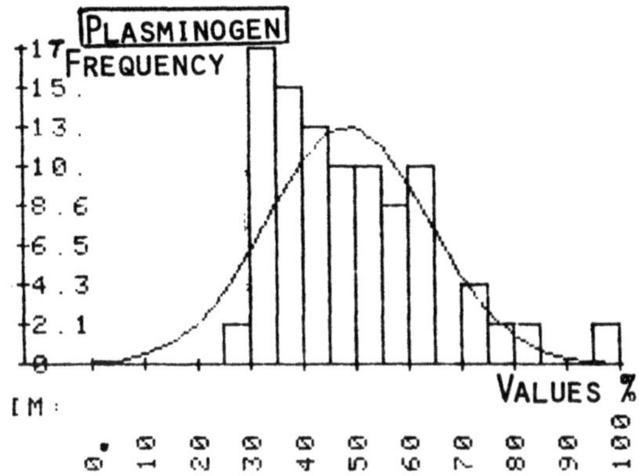

Fig. 4 : Plasmatic plasminogen values in patients with liver cirrhosis

but the half life is shortened with a normal turn over (61). The α2 fast antiplasmin lever (2) and consequently the α2 fast antiplasmin/plasminogen ratio are generally low (fig. 5).

This lack of balance can explain the high sensibility of these patients to activators and consequently to nicotinic acid. However, such an anomaly is rarely responsible for serious bleeding because systemic fibrinolysis needs the presence of fibrin. However, the phenomen may occur after the transfusion of partially coagulated or badly filtered products(7). This can also explain the disorder after a Le Veen shunts intervention. We can suggest a treatment with epsilon amino-caproic acid (or other similar molecules) in patients chronic bleeding. We used it sucessfully several times,apart from any associated pathology, transfusion and surgical intervention and in the absence of evident signs of coagulopathy. Indeed, in case of intravascular disseminated coagulation, anti-activators could stop the secondary fibrinolysis and thus, they could favour the deposits of fibrin in several organs and particularly in the kidney. Inhibitors such as α2 macroglobulin or α1 antitrypsin often increase in these patients but the physiological part of these inhibitors in fibrinolysis remains questionnable. The α2 rich glycoprotein in also reduced. It might interfere in fibrinolysis as an inhibitor, with α2 fast antiplasmin (55,78).

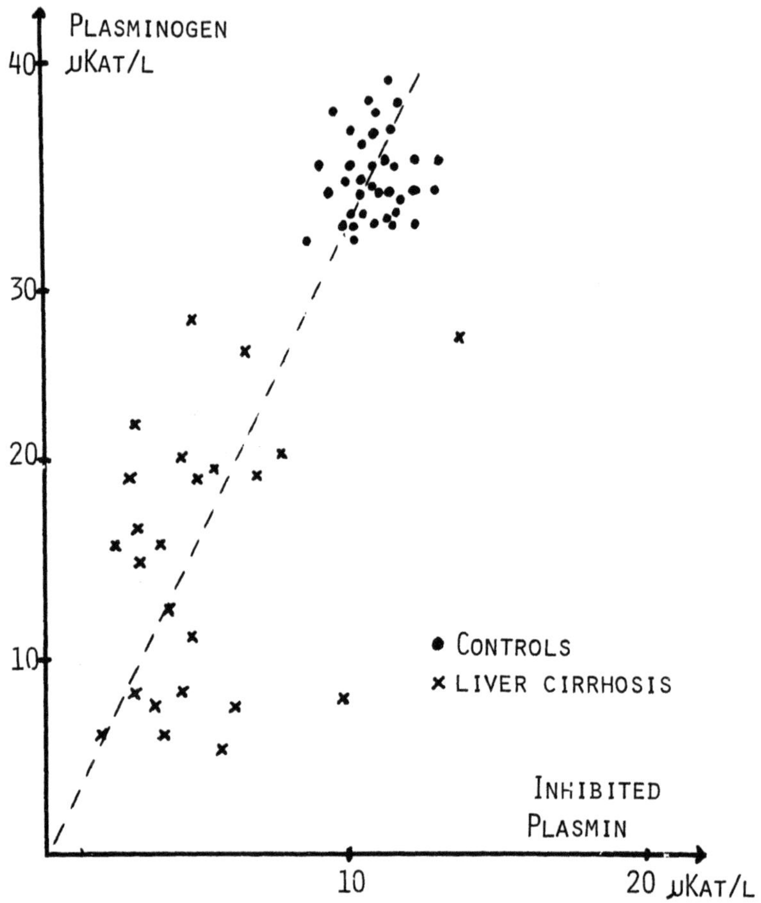

Fig. 5 : Correlations between α2 FAB and plasminogen in patients with liver cirrhosis.

4.3 Secondary to disseminated coagulation

The fibrinolytic response in chronic disease is generally moderate and it is often followed by the presence of fibrin degradation products. Treatment with heparin can stop this phenomen. However, fibrinolysis is important in acute disease, such as after a Le Veen shunts. In acute disorders, substitution is necessary and antithrombin III substitute seems to be more efficient particularly before the Leveen shunt intervention and during the first following days. The stabilisation of the coagulation system prevents any specific treatment of fibrinolysis, which can be even dangerous in favoring the intravascular deposits of fibrin. We unsucessfully tried to inject Künitz inhibitor in 3 patients with severe disseminated intravascular coagulation, following an injection of concentrated ascitis with an important secondary fibrinolysis.

4.4 Digestive activators and local digestive fibrinolysis.

The digestive mucosa and particularly the oesophageal and gastric mucosa have a fibrinolytic activity. This activity increases in cirrhotic patients (25,62). Such an increase can be responsible for some gastro-intestinal bleeding which are not explained by plasmatic coagulation anomalies, thrombocytopenia or systemic fibrinolysis. In such conditions, the local administration of epsilon-aminocaproic acid might be suggested. Yet such a therapy has to be carefully employed because of its possible absorption. These patients will simulteously receive transfusions which can lead to a coagulopathy.

This fibrinolytic hyperactivity of the mucosa can lead to an increase of the circulating activators. These activators go through circulation, especially if a local pression exists which can occur during the compression poke (26).

5. THE ABNORMALITIES OF PLATELETS.

Thrombocytopenia of the most common anomaly, due to splenic sequestration rather than to a coagulopathy (3,41,69,88). Toxic medullar disorders are excluded in this study (9). The place of platelet transfusion is difficult to precise: thrombocytopenia rarely leads to bleeding and the bleeding time is generally normal : the platelets numeration is not correlated with a haemorrhagic tendency (83). Apart from acute evolutions, chronic coagulopathy needs no platelet concentrates. Splenic sequestration makes platelet transfusions temporarily effective; that is the reason why it must be reserved to thrombocytopenia under $60.10^9/1$ with a serious haemorrhagic syndrom.

Thrombopathy has been described more recently. An abnormal response to ADP (5) and to thrombin (87) is observed, apart from the other coagulation abnormalities (5). Adhesion is also disturbed and these anomalies are correlated to the severity of the disease (24, 47, 77). Aggregation to ristocetin is also decreased perhaps because of a defect in glycoprotein I (63). Platelet transfusions should be made with precaution in case of serious haemorrhage. Platelet concentrates must be as fresh as possible because the products of platelet lysis such as phospholipids or PF4 can lead to hypercoagulability. Finally, a rapid immunisation in cirrhotic patients can lead to inefficacy of platelet transfusions or to "shiver and hyperthermia reaction" after non deleucocyted and no deplateled erythrocyte concentrates". In liver cirrhosis, an excess of ligh platelet population exists in Percoll isopycnic gradients. This significant increase is associated with a higher mean platelets volume (table 5).

	Normal	Cirrhosis
N	20	18
Mean vol.	8±20	10,6 ±2,2
Platelets distrib. index	9,7±1	10,6 ±0,36
F_1 (%)	19,6±3,3	48,5 ±14,5
F_2 (%)	33,6±5,4	35,1 ±9,9
F_3 (%)	46,4±6,9	16,16±6,1

Table 5 : Platelets density populations heterogeneity in liver cirrhosis (separations by Percoll isopycnic gradients).

We dit not find any correlation between the platelet density and plasminogen, prekallikrein and antithrombin III (fig 6).
The correlation with the platelet number seems to us to be poor. Probably the platelet abnormalities are not in relation with the liver synthesis disorders.

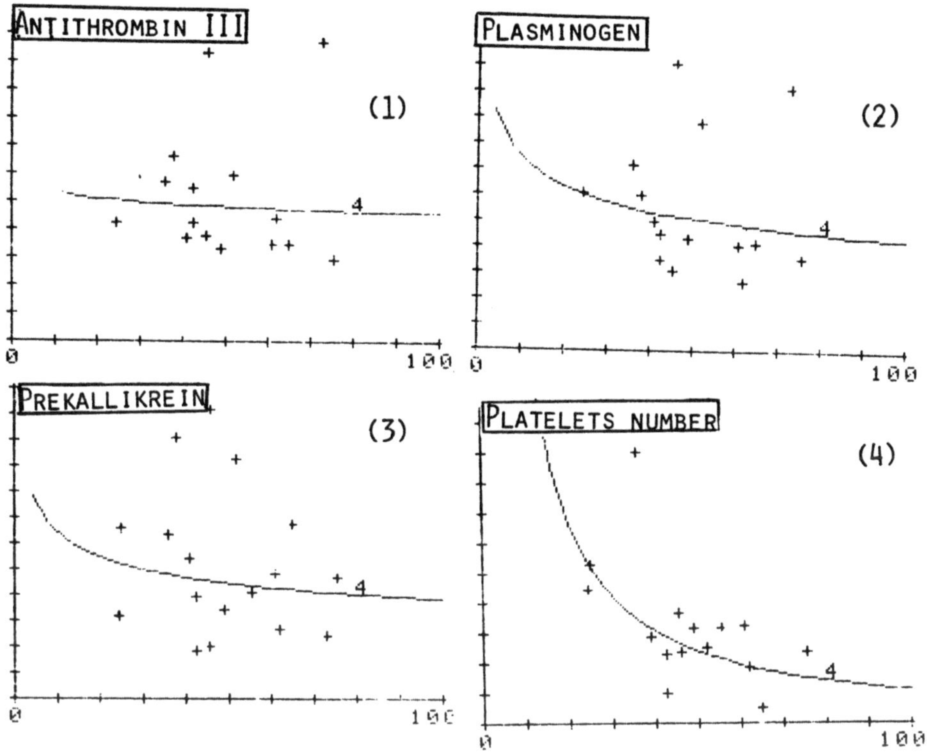

Fig. 6 : Correlations between light platelet populations in Percoll isopycnic gradients and antithrombin III (1), plasminogen (2), prekallikrein (3), platelets number (4).

6. THE INFLUENCE OF RED CELLS AND HEMOLYSIS.

Anisocytosis, schizocytosis, stomatocytosis and even acanthocytosis are frequently noticed in cirrhotic patients. Hemolytic reactions remain unusual but can lead to a coagulopathy (71). We think it is a good indication for heparinotherapy. Some of this hemolysis seems to be linked to abnormalities of the red cell membrane, which can explain their lack of filtrability in litterature (40). But our results are not in agreement with those of Hanss and Proff (table 6). In our study, the erythrocytes filtrability is not modified. On the contrary the deformability, tested by the Ektacytometer which is a new optical technique for measuring cell deformation in Couette flow) is increased/ This notion is also noticed by the low shear method : at γ 128,5 sec^{-1},

the viscosity is significantly decreased whatever hematocrit value. Clinical microcirculation disorders are not often observed. Thus, a transfusion of conserved red cells which have lost their properties of deformability can aggravate the situation.
Indeed, the ADP and 2-3 DPG levels rapidly correct in vivo, which is not the case for the red cell deformability (31).

	Normal	Cirrhosis
Filtrability (sec)	5,86±1,38	5,63±1,11
Deformability Ektacytometer	41,1±4,0	54,3±4,7
Viscosity mPa γ=128,5 sec^{-1}	4,06±0,2	3,63±0,88

Filtrability = Reid method
Deformability = erythrocytes ellipticity index

Table 6 : Rheological parameters modifications in liver cirrhosis

7. PORTAL HYPERTENSION

It is, especially with oesophagial varices, the prime cause of haemorrhage but the exact mechanism of haemorrhage remains questionnable.

7.1 Medical treatment.

Lysin vasopressin can be used as a visceral vasoconstrictor but it has many drawbracks : a short time of action, tachyphylactic and cardiotoxic effects. A local intra-arterial administration has been suggested but it cannot avoid the drawbacks entirely and it complicates the method. Triglycyl-lysin vasopressin slowly releases lysin vasopressin and does not present any toxic danger. It releases no plasminogen activators, contrary to lysin vasopressin (30,71,73). Such a release of activators can explain the return of haemorrhagic syndroms in patients depleted in fibrinolysis inhibitors. Recently, propanolol per os was suggested for a lowering of portal pressure in cirrhotics (fig. 7). Therefore, this product is mainly used as a preventive treatment (16). Although the number of the cases which have been published is still limited, the results are quite satisfactory(48,81) (table 7).

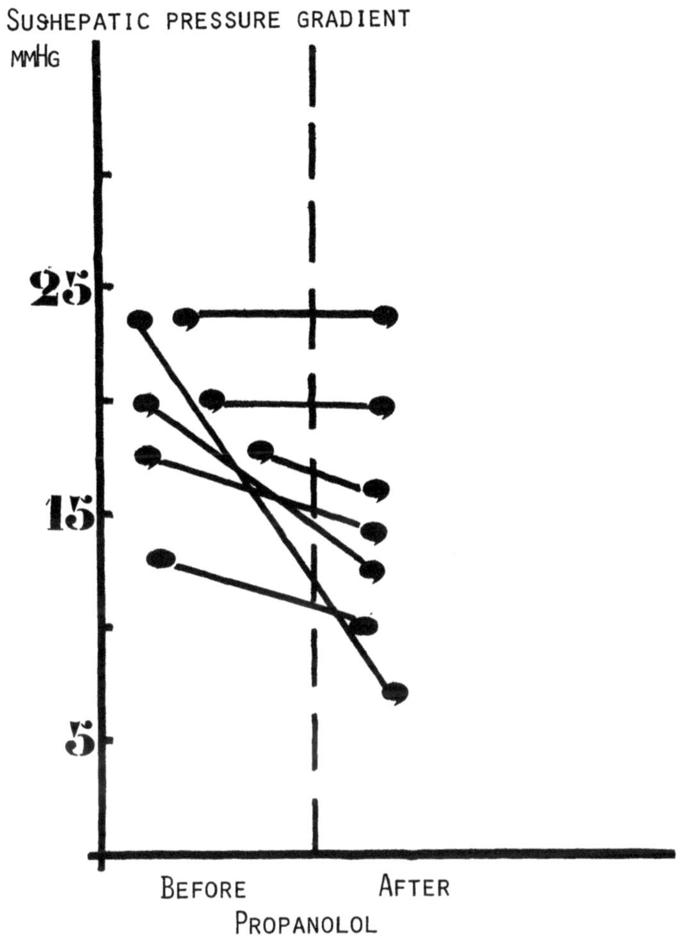

Fig. 7

	Patients	Haemorh. relapse	Death
>1 year	8	1	1
6 months<<1 year	4	1	0
TOTAL	12	2	1

Table 7 : Propanolol efficiency in haemorrhagical relapse prevention in liver cirrhoses (12 patients : 4 ♀, 8 ♂ 24-72 years old)

Its administration seems to stop bleeding during the transfusion. Prudence is required : propanolol is extracted from the liver and its accumulation in the organism of such patients can lead to encephalopathy and increase the pulmonary pressure (59). The interactions of these products with platelets remains questionnable but are negligible in a clinical point of view. Sclerosing injections are of a precious help and some authors suggest them in association with propanolol per os (17).

7.2 Surgical treatment

Many interventions have been suggested in order to reduce portal hypertension (6,64,67,68,72,98). Recently the peritoneojugular derivation (valve of Le Veen)happened to be effective in irreductible ascitis (10,52,66). However, this method leads to many complications and particularly to coagulopathy due to ascitis fluid re-injection (51,70,80,95). Antithrombin III substitution reduces, but does not totaly suppress that risk. Therefore the indications of this method must be limited. That is the reason why one of us (LEHN) perfected a simple method appropriate to patients who can not benefit from a Le Veen shunt(icterus, hepatitic coma, digestive haemorrhage, ascitic decompensation for more than one year). The schema nr 8 explains this method. The pump enables a controlled return of the ascitis liquid. Associated to the diet, the preparation consists in the administration of 15 000 units of heparin daily for a least 1 or 2 months (table 8). Any ascitis puncture is banished because of its infection risks and we have noticed an increase of fibrinogen in the ascitis after the punction. It seems to us that the fibrinogen is an important parameter in the fibrinolytic triggering after ascitic shunt.

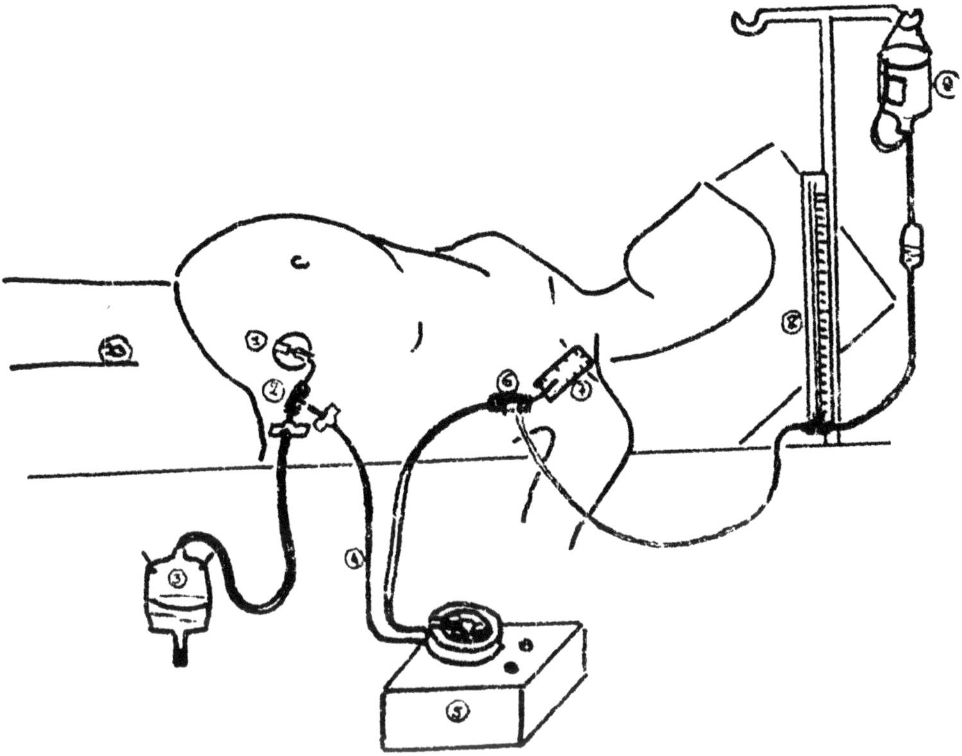

Shema 8 : method for ponction and continuous ascitis re-injection
(1) Silicon intraperitoneal catheter (cysto-cath)
(2) 3 ways tap
(3) bag for ascitis collection
(4) silicon line
(5) pump which permets to regulate the flow
(6) taps
(7) central catheter
(8) central venous pressure
(9) fluids
(10) urine collection.

Nr	shunt term	Results	Relapse	
1	6 d	±	after 1 month	digestive bleeding
2	3 d	-		hepatitic coma
3	10 d	+	d +12	death
4	6 d	±	partial	stable
5	6 d	±	+	Leveen sh. bleeding
6	19 d	+	partial at 1 month	stable
7	10 d	+	at 2 months	bleeding 3 months
8	5 d	+		stable 18 months
9	10 d	±	+	Snd sh. stable 6 months
10	10 d	±	+	Snd sh. stable 1 month

Table 8 : Clinical results after external shunt in 10 patients with ascitis by liver cirrhosis.

8. CONCLUSION

The treatment of bleeding disorders in patients with liver cirrhosis gives many problems. They are in relation with a bad comprehension of the physiopathological mechanisms . The symptomatic treatments risk to obtain incomplete results and often accidents. Recent studies have opened new ways where cooperative works are probably able to bring a rapid answer.

BIBLIOGRAPHY

1-AIACH M., ROGE J., BUSY M.F., DURAND H., GUEROULT N., CHANRION C. Dysfibrinogénémies acquises et affections hépatiques. A propos de 30 observations. Sem. höp. Paris, 1973,49 183.

2-AOKI O., YAMANAKA T. The $\alpha_2$plasmin inhibitor levels in liver diseases. Clin. Chim. Acta, 1978, 84, 99.

3-ASTER R.H. J. Clin. Invest., 1966, 45, 645.

4-AUROUSSEAU M.H., D'ANGELI J.L., JOSSO F. Antithrombin III versus prothrombin in liver cirrhosis, Haemostasis, 1981,10, 104.

5-BALLARD H.S., MARCUS A.J. Platelet aggregation in portal cirrhosis. Arch. Intern. Med., 1976, 136, 316.

6-BAUER J.J., GELERNT I.M., KREEL I. Portosystemic shunting in patients with primary biliary cirrhosis. A good risk disease. Ann. surgery, 1976, 183, 324.
7-BERGSTROM K., BLOMBACK B., KLEEN G. Studies on the plasma fibrinolytic activity in a case of liver cirrhosis. Acta med. Scand., 1960, 168, 291.
8-BICK R.L., SCHMALHORST W.R., SHANBROM E. Prothrombin complex concentrate : use in controlling the hemorrhagic dia thesis of chronic liver disease. Digestive diseases, 1975 20, 741.
9-BIGELOW F.S. Serotonin activity in blood ; measurements in normal subjects and in patient with thrombocytemia hemorrhagica and other hemarrhagic states. J. Lab. Clin. Med., 1954, 43, 759.
10-BISMUTH H., FRANCO D. La dérivation péritonéo-jugulaire dans l'ascite irréductible du cirrhotique. Nouv. press. méd., 1981, 10, 2707.
11-BLOMBACK B., CARLSON A., FRANZEN S., ZETTERQVIST E. Turn over of I-labelled fibrinogen in man. Studies in normal subjects, in congenital coagulation factor. Deficiency states, in liver cirrhosis, in polycythemia vera and in epidermolysis bullosa. Acta Med. Scand., 1966, 179, 557.
12-BLOOM A.L. Annotation, intravascular coagulation and the liver. Brit. J. Haemat., 1975, 30, 1.
13-BONEU B., SIE P., CARANOBE C., CASSIGNEUL J., PASCAL J. Progressive antithrombin activity and the concentration of three thrombin inhibitors in liver cirrhosis. Thromb. Haemost., 1982, 47, 78.
14-CASSILAS G., SIMONETTI C., PAVLOVSKY A. Chromatographic behavior of clotting factors. Brit. J. Haematol., 1969, 12, 363.
15-CEDERBAUM A.I., ROBERTS H.R. Complications of the use of prothrombin complex concentrates in liver disease. Clin. Res., 1973, 21, 92.
16-CHEVREL B. Le traitement médical des hémorragies de l' hypertension portale du cirrhotique par le Propanolol. M.C.D., 1982, 11, 69.
17-CLARK A.W., WESTABY D., SILK D.B., DAWSON J.L., MC DOUGALL B.R.D., MITCHELL K.J., STRUNIN L., WILLIAM S.R. Prospective controlled trial of injection sclerotherapy in patients with cirrhosis and recent variceal haemorrhage. Lancet, 1980, 2, 552.
18-COCCHERI S., MANNUCCI M., PALARETI G., GERVASONI W., POGGI M., VIGANO S. Significance of plasma fibrinopeptid A and high molecular weight fibrinogen in patients with liver cirrhosis. Brit. J. Haemat., 1982, 52, 503.
19-COCCHERI S., PALARETTI G., DALMONTE P.R., POGGI M., BOGGIAN O. Investigation on intravascular coagulation in liver disease : soluble fibrin monomer complex in liver cirrhosis. Haemostasis, 1979, 8, 8.
20-COCCHERI S., PALARETTI G., POGGI M., GRAUSO F Fibrin formation in liver cirrhosis : acquired dysfibrinogenemia or hampered polymerisation. Thromb. Haemost., 1979, 42, 536.
21- COLEMAN M., BETTIGOLD R.E., ANDERSON K.E., MAYER K., RYAN G.M. Fibrinogen survival in cirrhosis : effects of low dose heparin. Clin. Res., 1972, 20, 482.

22-COLEMAN M., FINLAYSON N., BETTIGOLE R.E., SADULA D., PASMANTIER M. Fibrinogen survival in cirrhosis : improvement by low dose heparin. Ann. intern. Med., 1975, 83, 79.
23-COLLEN D., ROUVIER J., CHAMONE A.F., VERSTRAETE M. Turnover of radiolabelled plasminogen and prothrombin in cirrhosis of the liver. Eur. J. Clin. Invest., 1978, 8, 185.
24-CORTET P., KLEPPING C., DEVANT J., LEBEL J.P., JACQUOT B. Le facteur plaquettaire au cours des cirrhoses alcooliques. Etude de l'adhésivité in vivo par le test de Borchgrevink. Arch. Mal. App. Digestif, 1964, 53, 73.
25-COX H.T., POLLER L., THOMSON J.M. Gastric fibrinolysis. A possible etiological link with peptic ulcer. Lancet, 1967, 1, 1300.
26-COX H.T., POLLER L., THOMSON J.M. Evidence for the release of gastric fibrinolytic activity into peripheral blood. Gut, 1969, 10, 104.
27-DAS P.C., CASH J.D. Brit. J. Haematol., 1969, 276, 1344.
28-DELMONT J., BISSET J., RAMPAL P., CAMOUS J.P., FAURE X. Métabolisme du fibrinogène chez le cirrhotique. Etude dynamique par méthode isotopique. Nouv. press. méd., 1976, 5, 1567.
29-DETTORI A.G., PONARI O., CIVARDI E., MEGHA A., PINI M., POTI R. Impaired fibrin formation in advanced cirrhosis. Haemostasis, 1977, 6, 137.
30-DOUGLAS J.G., FORREST J.A.H., PROWSE C.V., CASH J.D., FINLAYSON N.D.C. Effects of lysin vasopressin and glypressin on the fibrinolytic system in cirrhosis. Gut, 1979, 20, 565.
31- DROULLE C., ADJIZIAN J.C., BRISSART M.A., BARRE J., BLAISE A.M., PIGNON B., MASCRE M.W., POTRON G. A study of erythrocyte function in patients after multiple transfusions. Scand. J. Clin. Lab. Invest., 1981, 41, suppl. 156, 269.
32-DUCKERT F. Behaviour of antithrombin III in liver disease. Preliminary results. Scand. J. Gastroent., 1973, 8, suppl. 19, 109.
33-FISCHER M., FALKENSAMMER C., KLEIN H.J., IRSIGLER K., BRUNEDER H., SCHNACK H. Therapeutische Möglichkeiten bei Verbrauchskoagulopathien aktiver Leberzirrhosen : niederdosierte heparintherapie. W. klinis. Wochenschrift, 1976, 88, 488.
34-FLETCHER A.P., BIEDERMAN O., MOORE D. Abnormal plasminogen plasmin system activity (fibrinolysis) in patients with hepatic cirrhosis. Its cause and consequences. J. clin. Invest., 1964, 43, 681.
35-GIROLAMI A., PATRASSI G., CAPELLATO G., QUAINO V. An immunological study of prothrombin in liver cirrhosis. Blut, 1980, 41, 61.
36-GRAHN E.P., DIEZ A.A., STEFANIS S., DONNELLY W.J. Burr cells, hemolytic anemia and cirrhosis. Amer. J. Med., 1968, 45, 78.
37-GREEN G., DYMOCK I.W., POLLER L., THOMSON J.M. Use of factor VII rich prothrombin complex concentrates in liver disease. Lancet, 1975, 1, 1311.

38-GERRITS W.B.J., VAN AKEN W.G., VAN DER MEER J., VREEKEN J. Splenomegaly associated with chronic consumption coagulopathy. Acta med. Scand., 1974, 195, 425.
39-HAMILTON P.J., STALKER A.L., DOUGLAS A.S. Disseminated intravascular coagulation : a review. J. Clin. Pathol., 1978 31, 609.
40-HANSS M., PARAF A. Filtrabilité érythrocytaire et cirrhose Pathol. Biol., 1981, 29, 496.
41-HARKER L.A., FINCH C.A. Thrombokinetics in man. J. Clin. Invest., 1969, 48, 963.
42-HORDER M.H. Consumption coagulopathy in liver cirrhosis. Thromb. Diath. Haemorrhagica, 1969, suppl. 36, 313.
43-JOHANSSON S.A. Studies on blood coagulation factors in a case of liver cirrhosis. Acta med. Scand., 1964, 175, 177.
44-KASPER C.K. Postoperative thrombosis in hemophilia B. N. Engl. J. Med., 1973, 289, 160.
45-KWAAN H.C., MC FADZEAN A.J., COOK J. Lancet, 1956, 1, 132.
46-LANGIEWICZ J. Disturbances of haemostasis in liver cirrhosic patients treated with nicotinic acid. Rocz. AM Bialystok, 1977, 22, 193.
47-LANGLEY P.G., HUGUES R.D., WILLIAMS R. Platelet adhesiveness to glass beads in liver disease. Acta Haemat., 1982, 67, 124.
48-LEBREC D., POYNARD T., HILLON P., BENHAMOU J.P. Propanolol for prevention of recurrent gastro-intestinal bleeding. A controlled study. N. Engl. J. Med., 1981, 305, 1371.
49-LECHNER K., NIESSNER H., THALER E. Coagulation abnormalities in liver disease. Semin. Thromb. Hemost., 1977, 4, 40
50-LEGRE M., ARNAL J.C., GRATECOS N., TREFFOT M.J. Les grandes anémies hémolytiques au cours des cirrhoses. Etude des mécanismes et conséquences thérapeutiques avec rapport d' un cas. Ann. gastro-entérol. hépatol., 1977, 13, 539.
51-LERNER R.G., NELSON J.C., CORINES P., DEL GUERCIO L.R.M. Disseminated intravascular coagulation. Complication of Le veen peritoneovenous shunts. JAMA, 1978, 240, 2064.
52-LEVEEN H.H., CHRISTOUDIAS G., MOON I.P., LUFT R., FALK G. GROSBERG S. Peritoneovenous shunting for ascitis. Ann. Surg., 1974, 180, 580.
53-LEVY V.G., VERGOZ D., NAJMAN A., CAROLI J. Variations du taux de l'accélérine après splénectomie dans les cirrhoses Rev. Med. Chirur. des maladies du foie, 1968, 43, 3.
54-LEWIS J.H., DOYLE A.P. Effects of epsilon aminocaproic acid on coagulation and fibrinolytic mechanisms. JAMA, 1964, 188, 56.
55-LIJNEN H.R., JACOBS G., COLLEN D. Histidine-rich glycoprotein in a normal and a clinical population. Thromb. Res., 1981, 22, 519.
56-MANNUCCI M., MARI D. Hemostasis and liver disease. Haematologica, 1981, 66, 233.
57-MARASSI A., DI CARLO V., MANZULLO V., MANUCCI M. Thromboembolism following prothrombin complex concentrates and major surgery in severe liver disease. Thromb. Haemost., 1978, 39, 787.
58-MENACHE D., FAUVERT R., SOULIER J.P. Utilisation en hépato logie d'une fraction contenant la prothrombine, le comple-

xe proconvertine-facteur Stuart et le facteur antihémophilique B (P.P.B.). Path. Biol., 1959, 7, 2515.
59-NIES A.S., EVANS G.H., SHAND D.G. The hemodynamic effects of beta-adrenergic blockage on the flow dependent hepatic clearance of propanolol. J. of Pharmacology and experimen tal therapeutics, 1972, 184, 716.
60-NILSSON I.M., SJOERDSMA A., WALDENSTROM J. Antifibrinolytic activity and metabolism of E-aminocaproic acid in man Lancet, 1960, 1, 1322.
61-O'CONNEL R.A., GROSSI C.E., ROUSSELOT L.M. Role of inhibitors of fibrinolysis in hepatic cirrhosis. Lancet, 1964, 1 990.
62-OKA K., TANAKA K. Local fibrinolysis of oesophagus and stomach as a cause of hemarrhage in liver cirrhosis. Thromb. Res., 1979, 14, 837.
63-ORDINAS A., MARAGALL S., CASTILLO R., NURDEN A.T. A glycoprotein I defect in the platelets of three patients with severe cirrhosis of the liver. Thromb. Res., 1978, 13, 297
64-ORLOFF M.J., BELL R.H., HYDE P.V., SKIVOLOCKI W.P. Long term results of emergency portacaval shunt of bleeding oesophageal varices in a selected patients with alcoholic cirrhosis. Ann. Surg., 1980, 192, 325.
65-PALASCAK J.E., MARTINEZ J. Dysfibrinogenemia associated with liver disease. J. Clin. Invest., 1977, 60, 89.
66-PALIARD P., PARTENSKY C., SAUBIER E. Ascite "irréductible" du cirrhotique. Résultat de la dérivation péritonéo-jugulaire chez 16 malades. Nouv. Press. Med., 1981, 10, 2715.
67-PERA C., VISA J., RODES J., TERES J., TRIAS M., LATRE M.L. GRANDE L. Anastomose spléno-rénale préférentielle par voie rétro-péritonéale. Schweiz. Rundschau Med. (PRAXIS), 1980, 69, 128.
68-PEREIRAS R., VIAMONTE M., RUSSEL E., LEPAGE J., WHITE P., HUTSON D. New techniques for interruption of gastro-oesophageal venous blood flow. Diagnostic radiology, 1977, 124 313.
69-PENNY R., ROZENBERG M.C., FIRKIN B.G. Blood, 1966, 27, 1.
70-PHILIPS L.L., RODGERS J.B. Procoagulant activity of ascitic fluid in hepatic cirrhosis : in vivo and in vitro. Surgery 1979, 86, 714.
71-PHILIPPE P., DECAMPS A., MARCHEIX J.C., MARQUES-VERDIER A. Acanthocytose, grande hémolyse et coagulation intravasculaire disséminée au cours d'une cirrhose éthylique. Nouv. Press. Méd., 1979, 8, 3553.
72-PRANDHI D., RUEFF B., ROCHE-SICOT J., SICOT C., MAILLARD J.N., BENHAMOU J.P., FAUVERT T. Life-treatening hemorrhage of the digestive tract in cirrhotic patients. Amer. J. Surgery, 1976, 131, 204.
73-PROWSE C.V., DOUGLAS J.E., FORREST J.A.H., FORSLING M.L., FORSLING M.L. Haemostatic effects of lysin vasopressin and triglycyl lysin vasopressin infusion in patients with cirrhosis. Europ. J. of Clin. Invest., 1980, 10, 49.
74-RAKE M.O., FLUTE P.T., PANNELL G., WILLIAMS R. Intravascular coagulation in acute hepatic necrosis, Lancet,1970,1,533.

75-RAKE M.O., SHILKIN K.B., WINCH J., FLUTE P.T., LEWIS M.L. WILLIAMS R. Early and intensive therapy of intravascular coagulation in acute liver failure. Lancet, 1971, 2, 1215.
76-ROBERTSON B.R. Effect of nicotinic acid on fibrinolytic activity in health, in thrombotic disease and in liver cirrhosis. Acta Chir. Scand., 1971, 137, 643.
77-RUBIN M.H., WESTON M.J., LANGLEY P.G., WHITE Y., WILLIAMS R. Platelet function in chronic liver disease. Relationship to disease severity. Digestive diseases and Sciences 1979, 24, 197.
78-SAITO H., GOODNOUGH L.T., BOYLE J.M. Reduced histidine-rich glycoprotein levels in plasma of patients with advanced liver cirrhosis. Amer. J. Med., 1982, 73, 179.
79-SCHIPPER H.G., TEN CATE J.W. Antithrombin III transfusion in patients with hepatic cirrhosis. Brit. J. Haemat., 1982 52, 25.
80-SCHWARTZ M.L., SWAIN W.R., VOGEL S.B. Coagulopathy following peritoneovenous shunting. Surgery, 1979, 85, 671.
81-SOGAARD P.E. Propanolol in portal hypertension. Lancet, 1981, 1, 1204.
82-SORIA J., SORIA C., SAMAMA M., COUPIER J., GIRARD M.L., BOUSSER J., BILSKI-PASQUIER G. Dysfibrinogénémies acquises dans les atteintes hépatiques sévères. Coagulation, 1970, 3, 37.
83-SPECTOR I., CORN M. Laboratory tests of hemostasis. The relationship to hemorrhage in liver disease. Arch. Intern. Med., 1967, 119, 577.
84-SPECTOR I., CORN M., TICKTIN H.E. Effect of plasma transfusions on the prothrombin time and clotting factors in liver disease. N. Engl. J. Med., 1966, 10, 1032.
85-STAUB P.W. Diffuse intravascular coagulation in liver disease. Semin. in Thromb. and Haemost., 1977, 4, 1.
86-STEIN S.F., HARKER L.A. Kinetic and functional studies of platelets, fibrinogen and plasminogen in patients with hepatic cirrhosis. J. Clin. Lab. Med., 1982, 99, 217.
87-THOMAS D.P., REAM J.V., STUART R.K. Platelet aggregation in patients with Laennec's cirrhosis of the liver. N. Engl J. Med., 1967, 276, 1344.
88-TOGHILL P.J., GREEN S., FERGUSON R. Platelets dynamics in chronic liver disease with special reference to the role of the spleen. J. Clin. Pathol., 1977, 30, 367.
89-TULLIS J.L., MELIN M., JURIDIAN P. Clinical use of human prothrombin complexes. N. Engl. J. Med., 1965, 273, 667.
90-TYTGAT G.N., COLLEN D.J., DE VREKER R.A. La diathèse hémorragique en cas de cirrhose du foie. Nouv. Rev. fr. Hémat., 1968, 40, 265.
91-TYTGAT G.N., COLLEN D., VERSTRAETE M. Metabolism of fibrinogen in cirrhosis of the liver. J. Clin. Invest., 1971, 50, 1690.
92-VERGOZ D., LEVY V.G., NAJMAN A., CAROLI J. Variations du facteur V au cours des splénectimies dans les cirrhoses. Rev. fr. études clin. et biol., 1967, 12, 725.
93-VERSTRAETE M., VERMYLEN J., COLLEN D. Intravascular coagulation in liver disease. Annual Review of Medicine, 1974,

25, 447.
94-VERSTRAETE M., VERMYLEN G., VERMYLEN J. Excessive consumption of blood coagulation components as a cause of hemorrhagic diathesis. Amer. J. Med., 1965, 38, 899.
95-VIALLET A., VILLENEUVE J.P. Intravascular coagulation and ascitic fluid infusion. Ann. Intern. Med., 1979, 91, 318.
96-WEINER M. The fibrinolytic response to nicotonic acid in abnormal liver states. Amer. J. Med. Science, 1963, 74, 294.
97-WILKINSON S.P. Endotoxin and liver disease. Scand. J. Gastroenterol., 1977, 12, 385.
98-YAMAMOTO S., HIDEMURA R., SAWADA M., TAKESHIGE K., IWATSUKI S. The late results of terminal oesophagoproximal gastrectomy (TEPG) with extensive devascularisation and splenectomy for bleeding oesophageal varices in cirrhosis. Surgery, 1976, 80, 106.
99-ZETTERQVIST E., VON FRANCKEN I. Coagulation disturbances with manifest bleeding in extrahepatic portal hypertension and in liver cirrhosis. Acta Med. Scand., 1963, 173, 753.

TREATMENT OF BLEEDING BY METHODS NOT DIRECTLY RELATED TO HAEMOSTASIS

P. REDING

1. INTRODUCTION

The clinician's attitude concerning bleeding in patients with liver disease is aimed to stop the bleeding and to restore the blood volume. The deficiency in haemostasis is a phenomenon which parallels the severety of the liver disease and which may aggravate the bleeding.

We would like to recall the commonly accepted attitudes for the treatment of acute upper gastrointestinal bleeding which is the greatest threat for the patient with liver disease.

2. ACUTE UPPER GASTROINTESTINAL BLEEDING.

Haematemesis and/or melaena are the prominent symptoms of acute upper gastrointestinal bleeding.

2.1 Emergency treatment

The goals of treatment are to maintain circulation (check heart rate, blood pressure and central venous pressure). Therefore, a large venous catheter should be inserted and fluid infusion with saline or macromolecules started as soon as blood has been withdrawn for typing, cross-matching, PTT, BUN, platelet count, haematocrit and red blood cells count. If necessary blood transfusion is started without delay. If the prothrombin time is prolonged, the patient is given fresh blood or packed cells with fresh frozen plasma. Banked blood may aggravate encephalopathy associated with gastrointestinal bleeding : as the longer blood is in storage in blood banks, the higher its ammonia content will be. The rate of transfusion should be governed by the clinical status of the patient and not by the haematocrit value. In the case of cirrhosis, it has been demonstrated that portal pressure can b decreased by lowering blood viscosity. Blood viscosity is decreased by an isovolumic hemodilution : that means correcting volume without giving red cells and therefore decreasing the haematocrit value. A haematocrit value of 30 % is an adequate value for tissue oxygenation and gives a lower viscosity to blood (9).

A large bore nasogastric tube is helpful because it confirms the diagnosis of upper G.I. bleeding (suction of bloo it clears the stomach and it helps to wash it with clear tap water before endoscopy.

Endoscopy will be performed as "early" as possible and will show precisely the site of bleeding in 90 % of cases.

2.2 Specific treatment according to endoscopic findings.

In liver diseases, bleeding is most often due to varices or acute mucosal damage. According to Franco, bleeding originates from varices in 52.4 % of the cases, from acute muc sal damage in 40.5 % of the cases and from a chronic peptic ul in 7.I % of the cases (4), while for Williams, most patients w portal hypertension and upper G.I. bleeding are in fact bleedi from ruptured varices.

Some studies have implicated gastric erosions as a major source of bleeding (3, I3). Those gastric erosions seem to be part of the portal hypertension disease, as the risk of bleeding from gastric erosions is higher in patients with large esophageal varices than in those with small varices or none (7) Moreover, they disappear after shunting procedures or are prevented from bleeding by propranolol treatment.

2.2.1 Bleeding varices. If the hemorrhage originates from esophageal or gastric varices, a nasogastric tube seems useless or even detrimental. Cimetidine does not stop bleedin and does not prevent recurrent variceal hemorrhage (IO). This publication adds evidence for the explosion theory (the cause bleeding is portal hypertension) rather than the erosion theory (the cause of bleeding is an erosion of the varix due to reflux of gastric acid). Intravenous vasopressin infusion at a rate of 0.4 U/min is a simple way to control hemorrhage and is considered to be the first line of treatment (I4). Vasopressin is a potent splanchnic vasoconstrictor that has major side effects mostly for the patient with myocardial damage. Somatostatin has less adverse effects but is also less potent than vasopressin and therefore is not recommended (2, I5, I2). Oral nitroglycerin as a venodilatator, can improve the hemodynamic response to vasopressin and further decrease the portal pressure. If vasopressin does not control bleeding, then balloon compression should be used. When control is obtained, mesenteric angiography is performed to check the patency of the portal vein and to study the portal system anatomy if an urgent surgery should be necessary.

If, despite temporary control, bleeding recurs, depending upon the local competences and experiences, the endoscopist for endoscopic sclerotherapy, or the radiologist for embolization of varices, or the surgeon (P-C shunt, Warren's shunt, stapple gun...) may be required. Long term control of bleeding from varices may be obtained by definitive surgery (suggested for class Child A and B), or endoscopic sclerotherapy. In two recent controlled trials, it has been shown, that with endoscopic sclerotherapy, bleeding can be controlled and the frequency of hemorrhage reduced, so far without significantly decreasing mortality (I7, I). In the prevention of recurrent gastrointestinal bleeding in patients with cirrhosis, propranolol has also been shown effective in one controlled trial (8). It acts by lowering the portal pressure by a decrease of cardiac output. Nevertheless, other controlled trials are urgently needed to compare surgery, endoscopic sclerotherapy, propranolol, or no treatment at all. The following table reports the results obtained by these different methods in the so-far published studies.

Table 1. Treatments of bleeding varices.

	N	Control HH %	Recur-rence	Mortality after procedure	Complic. Major	% Minor
Vasoconstriction	347	58	48	50	I7	3
Oesophageal tamponnade	784	77	46	5I	I6	5
Endoscopic sclerosis	452	85	29	24	7	I
Percutaneous obliteration	2I5	78	43	35	I5	3
Stapple gun	38	95	I7	39	I6	0
PC shunts	587	96	3	40	38	24

2.2.2 Ulcer or erosions. This chapter deals with chronic peptic ulcer, stress ulcer, and diffuse mucosal damage (exulcerations and erosions). As previously written, gastric erosions may be part of the portal hypertension spectrum of disease. Nevertheless, in case of bleeding from acute erosions, stress factors should be searched for and corrected, especially septicemia which is particularly frequent in patients with severe liver disease.

No controlled study exists to prove the efficiency of antacids or H_2 antagonists to stop bleeding from focal or diffuse lesions. However H_2 antagonists should be used because the can prevent further bleeding and they contribute to the healing of chronic gastric and duodenal peptic ulcers (1).

Prostaglandins, by their cytoprotective action, are still under experiment. In a controlled trial performed in patients bleeding from peptic ulcer, somatostatin (infusion of 250 ug/hour for 48 to I20 hours after an IV bolus of 250 ug) was shown to be effective in controlling 8 bleeding episodes out of IO (6).

There also exists different invasive but non surgical techniques to control bleeding. These would be used depending upon the availability and experience of the local team. The include intra-arterial infusion of vasopressin, selective embolization and endoscopic methods (bipolar electrocoagulation or laser). Surgery would be the last method to be considered, particularly for patients with persistent bleeding from ulcers, despite all the treatment mentioned above.

3.CONCLUSION

The treatment of acute upper G.I. bleeding in patients with liver disease, is aimed at stopping the bleeding from the ruptured varix, by acting on the factors thought to be responsible for the wall stress:1. By controlling portal hypertension by pharmacological (vasopressin, somatostatin, nitroglycerin) or surgical means (shunting procedures) 2. By counter-acting that hypertension : that is balloon compression 3. By thickening the varix wall : that is endoscopic sclerotherapy. Nevertheless despite all these measures, acute upper G.I. bleeding remains a deadful challenge as mortality has reached up to 48 % (I6).

REFERENCES

1. Bernuau J, Nouel O, Belghiti J, Rueff B. I98I. Severe upper gastrointestinal bleeding. Clinics in Gastroenterology, IO, 38 - 59.
2. Bosch J, Kravetz D, Rodes J. I98I. Effects of somatostatin on hepatic and systemic hemodynamics in patients with cirrhosis of the liver : comparison with vasopressin. Gastroenterology, 80, 5I8-525.
3. Dagradi AE, Mehler R, Ton DT. I970. Sources of upper gastrointestinal bleeding in patients with liver cirrhosis and large esophagogastric varices. Am. Journal of Gastroenterology, 54, 458-463.
4. Franco D, Durandy Y, Deporte A, Bismuth H. I977. Upper gastrointestinal haemorrhage in hepatic cirrhosis : causes and relation to hepatic failure and stress. Lancet I, 2I8-220.
5. Groszman RJ, Kravets D, Bosch J, Glickman M, Bruix J, Bredfeldt J, Conn HO, Rodes J, Storer EH. I982. Nitroglycerin improves the hemodynamic response to vasopressin in portal hypertension. Hepatology, 2, 757 - 762.
6. Kayasseh L, Gyr K, Keller U, Stelder GA, Wall M. I980. Somatostatin and cimetidine in peptic-ulcer hemorrhage - A randomized controlled trial. Lancet I, 844 - 846.
7. Lebrec D, De Fleury P, Rueff B, Nahum H, Benhamou JP. I980. Portal hypertension size of esophageal varices and risk of gastrointestinal bleeding in alcoholic cirrhosis. Gastroenterology, 9, II39-II44.

8. Lebrec D, Poynard T, Hillon P, Benhamou JP. I98I. Propranolol for prevention of recurrent gastrointestinal bleeding in patients with cirrhosis. A controlled study. N. Engl. Med. 305, I37I-I374.
9. Leveen HH, Ip M, Ahmed N, Mascardo T, Guinto RB, Falk G. I980. Lowering blood viscosity to overcome vascular resistance. Surg. Gyn. Obst. I50, I39-I49.
IO. Macdougall BRD, Williams R. I983. A controlled trial of cimetidine in the recurrence of variceal hemorrhage : implications about the pathogenesis of hemorrhage. Hepatology. 3, 69 - 73.
II. Macdougall BRD, Westaby D, Theodossi A, Dawson JL, Williams R. I982. Increased long term survival in variceal hemorrhage using injection sclerotherapy : results of a controlled trial. Lancet I, I24 - I27.
I2. Naeije R, Hallemans R, Mols P, Melot C, Reding P. I982. Effects of vasopressin and somatostatin on hemodynamics and blood gases in patients with liver cirrhosis. Crit. Care Med. IO, 578 - 582.
I3. Palmer ED. I969. The vigorous diagnostic approach to upper gastrointestinal tract haemorrhage. Journal Am. Med. Association, 207, I477 - I480.
I4. Shaldon S, Sherlock S. I980. The use of vasopressin in the control of bleeding from esophageal varices. Lancet II, 222 - 225.
I5. Sonnenberg GE, Keller U, Perruchoud A, Burckhard D, Gyr K. I98I. Effect of somatostatin on splanchnic hemodynamics in patients with cirrhosis of the liver and in normal subjects. Gastroenterology 80, 526 - 532.
I6. Tabak C, Eugene J, Juler GL, Sarfeh IJ. I982. Upper gastrointestinal hemorrhage in cirrhosis : timing and indications for active intervention. Am. J. Gastroenterol. 77, 947 - 948.
I7. Terblanche J, Northover JMA, Bormann P, Kahn D, Silber W, Barbezat GO, Sellars S, Campbell JA, Saunders SJ. I979. A prospective controlled trial of sclerotherapy in the long term management of patients after esophageal variceal bleeding. Surg. Gynec. Obstet. I48, 323 - 333.

DISCUSSION LECTURE REDING

Mannucci I am somewhat worried about the education of sclerotherapy.

Fondu Indeed, these sclerotherapy is not without any danger, I agree completely with you. I should like to ask Dr. Reding's opinion about this formal therapy.

Reding Sclerotherapy has no role in an urgent situation. But it has a place to prevent further bleeding for patients, mostly I would suggest class C patients and reserve surgery for patients class A and B. The sclerotherapy has some complications. I have shown to you a percentage drop of 17 percent of major complications with sclerotherapy. I was not aware of hematologic complications after that. Remember also that after sclerotherapy you may have a dysfunction in the contraction of the oesophagus.

From the audience We are also using now sclerotherapy for about 3 years and we had indeed for about 15 or 16 percent of major troubles with sclerotherapy as you mentioned, but we did not yet have D.I.C. with sclerotherapy. The sclerosis of the oesophagus, can be overcome and it was no major complication in our series. However, all therapies of varices have their own draw backs and one can never predict for a single patient if, for example, a Le-Veen shunt will not produce extensive liver insufficiency, and coma etc. As you have shown very well, mortality from these type of operations is very high. But it is successful, it is the best one. But the risk is very high.

STRATEGIES FOR RATIONAL HAEMOTHERAPY

R. MASURE

A rational haemotherapy, consists, in giving all the needed blood components in suitable amounts, avoiding degraded products and undesirable contaminants, avoiding too, the wastage of unneeded components, useful for other patients, considering the ethic aspect of human blood donation and the logistic problems of blood transfusion services.

The components necessary for therapy of bleeding in liver disease are diverse and variable. They might include :

1. For adequate haemostasis, fresh platelets, some or numerous coagulation factors, perhaps antithrombin III, protein C, α 2-antiplasmin and fibronectin.
2. In case of major blood loss, the priority should be to correct volaemia, before other substitute therapy, in order to safeguard the maximal integrity of the remaining healthy hepatocytes. For this reason, cristalloid or colloid plasma substitutes, combined with albumin or plasma protein solutions should be used in emergencies, supplemented if required, with red cells to ensure an adequate oxigen transport capacity of the circulation.

For adequate haemostasis, one can remember that the minimal concentrations of diverse components vary between 2 and 30 % of the normal level, according to the products and to the medical conditions. Another aspect is that the half disappearance times in vivo of different components vary between 4-5 hours and 4-7 days.

Furthermore, the degree of the deficiences and their mechanism change from patient to patient. It is therefore clearly evident that the substitutive therapy has to be carefully adapted to the individual situation.

Great deficiences of factors II, VII and X, being usually concerned, the use of concentrates of these factors is highly debated in hepatic failure. Four types of so called "Prothrombin complex" or Factor IX concentrates, commonly used for the treatment of haemophilia B, are available. However, the amounts of factors II and VII of these concentrates, vary largely according to the method of production (2) :

1. Some products contain substantial amounts of the four common vitamin-K dependant factors, as PPSB and Konyne.
2. Other concentrates have low amounts of factor VII, one of the most deficient factor in liver disease (Bebulin®, Defix®, Preconativ®, Prothromplex®, Supernine...).
3. Another product has low prothrombin content (Proplex®)
4. Lastly some concentrates have a high content of activated factors, particularly contra-indicated in hepatic failure, (Autoplex®, Feiba®).

The low content of a number of Factor IX concentrates in factor VII leaded to the production of a Factor VII concentrate in the United Kingdom (England, Scotland) and in Austria.

The factor IX concentrate available in the Belgian Red Cross Transfusion Centres, contains the 4 factors, the most used dose of 1000 units, bringing practically 1000 to 1200 units of factor IX, an amount slightly lower of factor X and II, and for factor VII about two-thirds of the amount of factor IX.

One may not forget that the rising rate in vivo of factors II, VII, IX and X, is reduced in relation with their relatively low molecular weight and their extravascular diffusion. The observed rise is calculated by using the proportion given amount in units against body weight, with a coefficient of a mean value of 1, the value varying between 0.4 and I.8, according to the patients and to the concentrates.

The use of this type of concentrate in patients with liver disease is debated for two main reasons : 1) risk of hepatitis B or non-A non-B virus transmission; 2) risk of diffuse intravascular coagulation in relation with the presence of activated clotting factors in some preparations.

The risk of hepatitis may be decreased by : 1) selecting carefully the donors, 2) non-remunerating donation in order to prevent dissimulations of pathology, 3) selecting the country of origin, 4) limiting the number of donations per batch (pool size), 5) pre-treating the plasma or the concentrate in order to inactivate or eliminate virus (ultra-violet light, bêta-propiolactone, extensive washing of DEAE-Sephadex before elution, selective PEG-precipitation from the eluate, heating).

Various "in vitro" and "in vivo" assays have been developped for detection of potential thrombogenicity of the concentrates. Several tests are used. None of them can be recommanded as a single screening test for quality control (2).

Factor IX concentrates are therefore not to be advised in acquired deficiences due to severe hepatic failure.

Factor VIII concentrates are sometimes used in severe hepatic failure with disseminated intravascular coagulation, particularly as cryoprecipitate, in order to bring at once factor VIII, fibrinogen and fibronectin. Purified concentrates have less fibrinogen and fibronectin, with higher risk of hepatitis.

Among blood components, the most used in treatment of bleeding from hepatic origin, are the following types of plasma :

- The freeze dried plasma finds here one of its rare actual indications, it is excellent source of factors II, VII, IX, X and fibrinogen, taking into account its possibility to be dissolved in half a volume of solvent when the infusion of large amount is needed without large increase of the volaemia.

- Fresh frozen plasma is in addition a good source of factor V and XI.
- Platelet rich plasma contains more than 80 milliard platelets per unit plasma.
- Platelet concentrates (more than 50 milliard per unit concentrate) is an unexpected source of blood coagulation factors, concentrated on their surface and in some granulations. It could be a very good treatment, if the repeated infusion of platelet concentrates did not quick in produce alloimmunization to platelet antigens.

It must be remembered that fresh frozen and platelet rich plasma contain anti-A and anti-B antibodies in opposition with the low isoagglutinin titers of freeze dried plasma.

Substitutive therapy for bleeding is not limited to coagulation or haemostasis factors. Hypovolaemia can contribute to the worsening of hepatic failure and disseminated intravascular coagulation.

It may be urgent and a priority, to correct this hypovolaemia with the first available products. The following therapeutic scheme has been recommended and found satisfactory (4) :

1. If the blood volume loss is equal or less than 20 %, infusion of saline, then colloid plasma substitute.
2. If the blood volume loss is between 20 and 35 %, increase colloid plasma substitute to 1 liter and then whole blood.
3. If the blood volume loss is over 35 %, associate albumine or other plasma protein solution, then blood.

Lundsgaard-Hansen has, in this manner, elaborated a basic diagram of blood component therapy, according to the values of hematocrit, total serum proteins, factors V and VIII and platelets, with the successive infusion of gelatin, red cell concentrates, stable plasma protein solution, fresh frozen plasma, and lastly, fresh whole blood (1).

The infusion of colloid plasma substitutes may however

enhance the haemostasis disorders and especially disseminated intravascular coagulation. This was observed in an experimental study, with simultaneous infusion of thrombin and of dextrans of various molecular weights, or gelatin, or stable plasma protein solution (3). Platelet number, platelet factor, 3 and 4, fibrinogen and antiplasmin activity, are more or less highly modified by substitutes alone, more with the infusion of thrombin, and still more with the association of both thrombin and substitutes. On the other hand, stable plasma protein solution appears devoid of any enhancing effect.

Whole blood versus red cell concentrate ? According to the basic diagrams of Lundsgaard-Hansen, red cell concentrate is given first, followed by fresh whole blood later on (1) :

1. Fresh whole blood, less than 6 hours old, has the advantage of supplying all the needed compounds, but only in amounts. The problem of the use of fresh blood is that of availability and of quality control (HBsAg, ALT,...).
2. Older whole blood has the disavantage of activation of platelets and of coagulation factors, and the increase of potassium.
3. Red cell concentrates offers a higher hematocrit rate (70 % against 30 % for whole blood), low amounts of activated platelets and activated coagulation factors, low amounts of potassium and of sodium citrate. The CPD anticoagulant solution maintains, in addition, their oxygen-carrying capacity, immediately available during their complete period of preservation.

Conclusion.

The adopted strategy aims at being efficient, safe and realistic. The choice of components, to the important specific needs has to be adapted. Therefore, adequate amounts on the necessary products need to be administered in a good sequence at the right moment.

REFERENCES

1. Lundsgaard-Hansen P. Component therapy of surgical hemorrhage : red cell concentrates, colloids and crystalloids. Biblthca Haemat. 46 : I47-I69, Karger, Basel, I980.
2. Masure R, Myllyla G, Temperley I, Stampfli K. Preparation and use of coagulation factors VIII and IX for transfusion. Co-ordinated blood transfusion research. Council of Europe, Strasbourg, I980, pp. I-96.
3. Moriau M, Rodhain J, Noël H, Masure R. Comparative effects of dextrans, gelatin and stable plasma protein solution (SPPS) on the experimental disseminated intravascular coagulation (DIC). Vox Sang. 27 : 4II-428, I974.
4. O'Riordan J.P, Aebischer M, Darnborough J, Thoren L. The indications for the use of albumin, plasma protein solutions and plasma substitutes. Co-ordinated blood transfusion research. Council of Europe, Strasbourg, I978, pp. I-77.

DISCUSSION LECTURE MASURE

Williams I would like to make -to my clinical feeling- a very important remark and to back Prof. Masure in the stragegy for the rationate of hemotherapy, is indeed to use very carefully blood and blood factors. Indeed, you must know that for non-A, non-B transfusion hepatitis although the mortality is not high and is something like 1/1000 having a liver coma out of the non-A, non-B; chronicity from non-A, non-B after transfusion is about 50 percent, is 1/2. If you consider the worse of the cases, which are not produced apparently by transfusion or contact with blood, this is only 15 percent and maybe this is due to some other virus because we don't know non-A, non-B virus is really totally unknown and several authors think that more viruses are in cause. But, nevertheless, whatever it may be, if you get it from blood, are the chances or risk for chronicity 50 percent and I should make a plea for eliminating all suspected donors with increased transaminase. There has been some rule that the transaminase should never be above 60 units. But I think this is a much too high figure and I should prefer to eliminate all elevations of transaminase, whatever they may be. And I think we are doing it here, we have a very long rate of post-transfusion non-A, non-B hepatitis. We have a rather high, and that's why I make a plea for this elimination, when blood is used we don't control tha fresh blood, neither for hepatitis antigen, neither for transaminase; than indeed, almost all cases we see of post-transfusion hepatitis are due to uncontrolled blood used as fresh blood in urgent situations.

AT-III CONCENTRATE TREATMENT: CURRENT EXPERIENCE

J.W. ten Cate, H.G. Schipper, H.R.Büller

Antithrombin-III is a major inhibitor of blood coagulation (1). Congenital deficiency states have been recognized in families with spontaneous thromboembolic episodes already at young age (2). The acquired deficiency state as for example occurring in liver cirrhosis is a much more frequently observed condition. Antithrombin-III (AT-III) is synthesized in the liver and its synthesis has also been shown to occur in cultured endothelial cells (3). Decreased synthesis is the main cause of AT-III deficiency in cirrhosis. Increased loss of AT-III in proteinuria (4) or in case of increased gastrointestinal loss in inflammatory bowel disease (5) may also lead to acquired AT-III deficiency and thromboembolic complications.

Severe liver cirrhosis is associated with a so called low grade diffuse intravascular coagulation as revealed by increased turnover of fibrinogen (6), prothrombin (7) and/of plasminogen (8).

This more or less steady state increased turnover is considered to be the result of continuous activation of the coagulation system by ill defined triggers, such as endotoxins or necrotic hepatocytes.

The AT-III plasma level is decreased, as a result the defense mechanism against activated clotting factors and subsequent fibrinogen consumption is also decreased.

In normal conditions AT-III forms 1:1 complexes with activated clotting factors (9) in order to prevent widespread fibrin deposition.

In conditions with low AT-III plasma levels this important inhibitory mechanism may fail with thromboembolic complications as a consequence.

In liver cirrhosis with an associated increased turnover of fibrinogen and decreased levels of AT-III , the situation is still compensated. When an additional triggering mechanism, i.e. surgery or sepsis, becomes operative decompensation may occur due to rapid exhaustion of AT-III. Decompensated diffuse intravascular coagulation is characterized by massive consumption of clotting factors, fibrinogen and/of platelets and fibrin deposition in all organ system with subsequent organ failure,

This situation is illustrated in the following case report (10).

CASE REPORT

A 54-year old man with liver cirrhosis was admitted with bleeding oesophageal varices. During observation bleeding recurred, the coagulation status deteriorated, blood cultures became positive for pseudomonas aeruginosa. His condition required urgent surgical interference, i.e. thoracotomy and ligation of the oesophageal varices. His coagulation status had therefore to be corrected in a short period of time. His coagulation profile revealed diffuse intravascular coagulation with massive consumption of fibrinogen, thrombocytopenia and a positive ethanol gelation test (table I).

TABLE I

Blood test	(1) 0 min	(2) 30 min	(3) 80 min	(4) 110 min	(Operation) 250 min	370 min	Normal values
AT-III (%)	37	64	67	97	82	86	80-140
Factor II (%)	44	52	78	78	75	120	90-150
Factor X (%)	48	59	92	81	100	120	80-140
Fibrinogen (mg/dl)	65	65	113	133	159	194	175-350
Platelets (x 10^9/1)	48	52	63	69	85	109	150-350
Ethanol-gelationtest	+ve	+ve	+ve	weakly +ve	-ve	-ve	-ve
Haematocrit (1/1)	0.23	0.26	0.26	0.26	0.28	0.38	0.37-0.47

Infusion of (1) 1650 U AT-III; (2) P.P.S.B. (20 donors); (3) 1650 U AT-III + 500 U heparin; (4) cryoprecipitate (20 donors), and platelets (8 donors).

In this situation the severe coagulation status was rapidly improved and the patient underwent uncomplicated surgery.

From these initial experiences using human AT-III concentrate (KabiVitrum, Stockholm, Sweden) we concluded that a systemic study in liver cirrhosis should be undertaken to evaluate the effect of human AT-III concentrate more precisely (11).

Therefore a study, approved by the scientific and medical ethical committees of our hospital, was undertaken in seven patients with liver cirrhosis.

Human AT-III concentrate in stable liver cirrhosis.

Liver cirrhosis, in 4 patients due to alcohol abuse, in 3 patients of unknown etiology, was biopsy proven.

The study design was:

Injection of 44-85 μCi ^{125}I-fibrinogen preceeded by hepatitis-B immunoglobulin i.m. and 500 mg potassium iodide orally which was continued for 14 days.

Regular blood specimen were taken to determine the kinetics of ^{125}I-fibrinogen and for other coagulation parameters.

Seven days after injection of ^{125}I-fibrinogen, transfusion was started with a single dose of human AT-III concentrate (1650-4400 U AT-III dissolved in pyrogen free distilled water), immediately followed by a continuous intravenous infusion of AT-III during 48 hours in order to obtain stable plasma levels of around IU/ml plasma.

We observed correction of increased ^{125}I-fibrinogen turnover towards normal levels upon this AT-III transfusion regimen in all patients (table II).

TABLE II

Metabolic parameters of ^{125}I-fibrinogen:

Parameter	decreased AT-III	corrected AT-III	Control group
Half life α_2	76 (± 14)	108 (± 19)	109 (±9)
k_{10}	53 (± 12)	77 (± 18)	85 (±4)

During this study occasional transient rises of platelet counts and of fibrinogen plasma levels were observed upon increasing AT-III plasma levels.

CONCLUSION: Correction of AT-III plasma levels in patients with stable liver cirrhosis appeared to interfere with the low grade (compensated) DIC as shown by the correction of ^{125}I-fibrinogen half lives to normal values.

Experimental studies in animals (12)

Although no effects of AT-III concentrates were observed on primary hemostasis, i.e. no prolongation of the bleeding times, a further study in animals was felt to be required. We used the rat bleeding model in rats described by Hobbelen (13) which implies a standard incision in the mm gluteii and quantitative measurement of blood loss by Hb determination for 30 minutes.

Prior to the incision the test compound was infused, which was either saline or human AT-III concentrate.

Increasing the plasma AT-III levels to 2 U/ml or even 8 U/ml had no effect on haemostasis in this model (table III).

TABLE III

Compound	N	Hb (%)	significance
Saline	24	100*	-
AT-III 2 U/ml	8	105	n.s.
AT-III 8 U/ml	8	98	n.s.

*The mean blood loss in control animals was arbitrarily expressed as 100 %.

It was interesting to observe that heparin administered in a low dose alone significantly increased the blood loss. This effect was even more pronounced at the highest AT-III plasma levels (table IV).

TABLE IV

	Mean blood loss relative to controls
Controls (n=24)	100%
Heparin* (n=8)	157% $p< 0.005$
AT-III 2 U/ml (n=8)*	166% $p< 0.005$
AT-III 8 U/ml (n=8)*	235% $p< 0.0001$

*Low dose heparin (0.25 mg/kg b.w.)

CONCLUSION: Increasing AT-III plasma levels to high concentrations relative to other clotting factors does not affect primary haemostasis.

This observation is more or less in agreement with our studies in liver cirrhosis patients. Relative high AT-III plasma levels when compared to the levels of other clotting factors did not affect bleeding times. Therefore these combined observations do suggest that transfusion of human AT-III concentrate is relatively safe in this respect.

Administration of heparin in addition should on the contrary be monitored very carefully. Unexpected impairment of haemostasis is then possible as revealed by our animal experiments.

LeVeen shunt study (14)

Due to our previous experiences we considered a prophylactic study using human AT-III concentrate in patients undergoing LeVeen shunt operation reasonable.

LeVeen shunt surgery in patients with liver cirrhosis for reasons of intractable ascites is complicated by shunt clotting, disseminated intravascular coagulation, fever and sepsis.
Also laboratory findings are suggestive of either mild to severe DIC. The latter is clinically associated with severe bleeding symptoms and was observed mainly in patients having severely decreased AT-III plasma levels prior to surgery.

AT-III deficiency obviously facilitates the occurrence of decompensated DIC which is assumed to be initiated by endotoxin - cellular components and/or activated clotting factors present in the ascites.

In this study five patients received AT-III concentrate in a bolus injection followed by continuous infusion in order to maintain the plasma levels at 1 U/ml. Prior to injection the patients received hepatitis B-immunoglobulin.

Despite this treatment DIC and bleeding occurred in 3 of 5 patients. Detailed coagulation studies revealed distinct fibrinogen and platelet consumption and positive ethanol gelation tests to occur in the course of this rigorous AT-III transfusion scheme.

CONCLUSION: Human AT-III concentrate transfusion alone does not prevent DIC and bleeding in the postsurgical period following LeVeen shunt implantation.

GENERAL CONCLUSIONS:

At present no clear indications for human-AT-III treatment have been revealed by clinical trials.

Some evidence for rational use in patients with severe AT-III deficiency and decompensated DIC has been provided.

Restrictions in the use of these concentrates are related to the complications observed using other factor concentrates such as hepatitis and the autoimmune deficiency syndrome.

REFERENCES

1. Abildgaard, U. In: Recent advances in blood coagulation, no 3, Ed. L. Poller., Churchill Livingstone, Edinburgh, 1981.

2. Egeberg, O., Inherited antithrombin deficiency causing thrombophilia. Thromb. Diath. Haem., 1965, 13: 516.

3. Chan, V. and T.K. Chan., Antithrombin III in fresh and cultured human endothelial cells: a natural anticoagulant for the vascular anticoagulant from the vascular endothelium. Thromb. Res., 1979, 15: 209.

4. Kauffman, R.H., J. de Graeff and G. Brutel de la Rivière. Unilateral thrombosis and nephrotic syndrome. Am. J. Med., 1976, 60: 1048.

5. Lake, A.M., J.Q. Stauffer, M.J. Stuart., Hemostatic alterations in inflammatory bowel disease. Dig. Dis., 1978, 23: 897.

6. Tytgat, G.N., D. Collen, M. Verstraete., Metabolism of fibrinogen in cirrhosis of the liver. J. Clin. Invest., 1971, 50: 1690.

7. Collen, D., J. Rouvier, D.A.F. Chamone, M. Verstraete., Turnover of radiolabeled plasminogen and prothrombin in cirrhosis of the liver. Eur. J. Clin. Invest., 1978, 8: 185.

8. Ibid.

9. Rosenberg, R.D. and P.S. Damus., The purification and mechanism of action of human antithrombin-heparin cofactor. J. Biol. Chem., 1973, 248: 6490.

10. Schipper, H.G., L.H. Kahlé, C.S.P. Jenkins, J.W. ten Cate., Antithrombin III transfusion in disseminated intravascular coagulation. Lancet, 1978, II: 854.

11. Schipper, H.G., and J.W. ten Cate.. Antithrombin-III transfusion in patients with liver cirrhosis. Brit. J. Haematol., 1982, 52: 25.

12. Büller, H.R., P.M.J. Hobbelen, A.W.N. Princen, H.C.T. Moelker, J.W. ten Cate., The effects of high plasma antithrombin III levels in the presence or absence of heparin on the bleeding tendency using an experimental model in rats. Thromb. Res., 1983, accepted for publication.

13. Meuleman, D.G., P.M.J. Hobbelen, G. van Dedem, H.C.T. Moelker., A novel antithrombotic heparinoid (:T: Org 10172) devoid of bleeding inducing capacity. Thromb. Res., 1982, 27: 353.

14. Antithrombin III infusion in patients undergoing peritoneovenous shunt operation: failure in the prevention of disseminated intravascular coagulation. Büller, H.R. and J.W. ten Cate., Thromb. Haem., 1983, in press.

DISCUSSION LECTURE TEN CATE

Fondu Are you convinced from statistical evidence that this fo of therapy is useful?

Ten Cate I am convinced that AT III substitution is useful. But when you give AT III maybe there is a danger to give hep

I N D E X

GPSR Compliance
The European Union's (EU) General Product Safety Regulation (GPSR) is a set of rules that requires consumer products to be safe and our obligations to ensure this.

If you have any concerns about our products, you can contact us on

ProductSafety@springernature.com

In case Publisher is established outside the EU, the EU authorized representative is:

Springer Nature Customer Service Center GmbH
Europaplatz 3
69115 Heidelberg, Germany

www.ingramcontent.com/pod-product-compliance
Ingram Content Group UK Ltd.
Pitfield, Milton Keynes, MK11 3LW, UK
UKHW020818290926
15470UKWH00003B/1236
9780898386400